Examination Notes f

Examination Notes for the MRCPsych Part I (New Syllabus)

B.K. Puri MA, MB, BChir, MRCPsych
Honorary Registrar in Psychiatry,
The Department of Psychiatry,
Addenbrooke's Hospital, Cambridge

J. Sklar LRCP, MRCS, MB BS, MRCPsych, AssMemBritPsychoanalSoc
Psychoanalyst and Consultant Psychotherapist,
The Department of Psychotherapy,
Addenbrooke's and Fulbourn Hospitals, Cambridge

With a Foreword by

Professor E.S. Paykel MD, FRCP, FRCPsych
Professor of Psychiatry,
University of Cambridge

Butterworths
London Boston Singapore Sydney Toronto Wellington

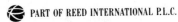 PART OF REED INTERNATIONAL P.L.C.

First published 1989

© Butterworth & Co. (Publishers) Ltd, 1989

British Library Cataloguing in Publication Data
Puri, B. K.
   Examination notes for the MRCPsych part I (New syllabus).
   I. Title   II. Sklar, J.
   616,89

   ISBN 0-407-01671-6

Library of Congress Cataloging in Publication Data
Puri, Basant K.
   Examination notes for the MRCPsych part I (new syllabus) / B.K.
Puri, J. Sklar : with a foreword by E.S. Paykel.
      p.   cm.
   Includes bibliographies and index.
   ISBN 0-407-01671-6 :
   1. Psychiatry—Examinations, questions, etc.   I. Sklar, J.
(Jonathan)   II. Title.
   [DNLM: 1. Psychiatry—examination questions. WM 18 P985e]
RC457.P869   1989
616.89'076—dc20
DNLM/DLC
for Library of Congress   89-15908
                                                                        CIP

Composition by Genesis Typesetting, Borough Green, Sevenoaks, Kent
Printed and bound by Hartnolls Ltd., Bodmin, Cornwall

Foreword

The MRCPsych examination has recently been given a revised
format. Part I, previously an examination in basic science, now
incorporates the fundamental clinical skills and knowledge which
should be acquired in the first year of psychiatric training.

Dr Basant Puri is a Cambridge graduate, sufficiently recently
trained in psychiatry to be well in touch with examination
requirements. He has published a volume of specimen multiple
choice questions for self-assessment for the MRCPsych Part 2. Dr
Sklar is Consultant Psychotherapist and Regional Tutor in
Psychotherapy in Cambridge. In the present volume the authors
summarize the factual knowledge needed for the Part I. The
contents reflect well the new balance between clinical and basic
elements. It is to be hoped that this book will help new psychiatric
trainees as they tackle the considerable demands of their first year.
I and the authors wish them well in their task.

E. S. Paykel
Professor of Psychiatry, University of Cambridge
June 1989

Preface

This book is aimed primarily at the needs of candidates for the MRCPsych Part I or equivalent examinations. The MRCPsych Part I is a revised examination which was introduced in October 1987, and which differs from the previous Preliminary Test of the MRCPsych. This book covers the main areas of the new syllabus, and overall aims at a holistic approach to psychiatry; the authors were interested in promoting a view of psychiatry that is both organically and psychodynamically determined. However, it is not intended to be a substitute for wider reading or practice in clerking patients. The latter is felt by the authors to be of paramount importance, and is indeed reflected in the approach of the new Part I examination. As Pierre Janet pointed out, the best textbook of psychiatry is the patient.

This book should also prove useful to medical students, psychiatric nurses, psychologists and trainee psychotherapists.

The syllabus used as the basis of the chapter contents is that given in the Eighth Revision of the *General Information and Regulations for the MRCPsych Examinations*[1]. The specimen multiple choice questions that appear in this book are based on those given in the *Working Party for Review of the MRCPsych Report to the Court of Electors*[2].

We should like to express our thanks to Professor E.S. Paykel for kindly providing a Foreword.

Cambridge 1989   B.P.
                                                                 J.S.

References

1. The Royal College of Psychiatrists (1987) *General Information and Regulations for the MRCPsych Examinations,* 8th revision. London: The Royal College of Psychiatrists.
2. The Royal College of Psychiatrists (1985) *Report to the Court of Electors, The Royal College of Psychiatrists Working Party for Review of the MRCPsych.* London: The Royal College of Psychiatrists.

Contents

Chapter 1

Neuroanatomy

Syllabus requirements

In neuroanatomy the candidate's knowledge of the brain and spinal cord and peripheral nervous system should be updated as the basis of neurological examination and diagnosis.

(The anatomy and physiology of the limbic system is part of the MRCPsych Part II syllabus.)

The neurone

A neurone or nerve cell consists of (see Figure 1.1):

- The perikaryon, neurocyte or cell body
- Neurites that project from the perikaryon, including:
  - the axon
    - usually one per neurone
    - originates from the axon hillock
    - Nissl substance absent
    - conducts impulses away from the perikaryon
    - myelin sheath always absent from initial segment
  - dendrites
    - usually more than one per neurone
    - Nissl substance present
    - some have dendritic spines
    - conduct information to the perikaryon

Classification

Morphological
- Unipolar
  - perikaryon has one neurite only which divides into two branches
  - e.g. in the posterior root ganglion

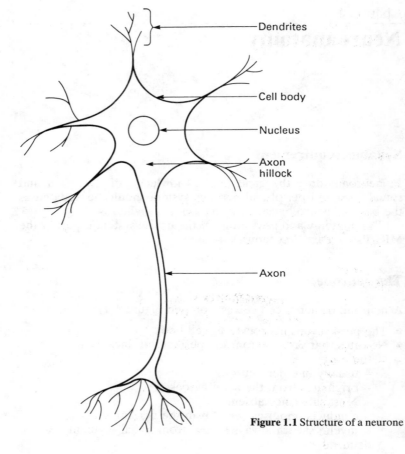

Figure 1.1 Structure of a neurone

- Bipolar
  - perikaryon has two neurites only
  - e.g. in the retina
- Multipolar
  - one axon and more than one dendrite
  - majority of neurones

By size
- Golgi type I
  - long axon
  - axons form the long fibre tracts of the CNS

○ axons form the nerve fibres of peripheral nerves
○ e.g. cortical pyramidal cells
• Golgi type II
○ short axon
○ much more numerous than Golgi type I neurones
○ e.g. abundant in the cerebral cortex

Neuronal structure

• Nucleus
○ relatively large
○ Barr body in females
○ usually one prominent nucleolus
• Cytoplasm
○ contains Nissl substance, Golgi apparatus, mitochondria, microfilaments, microtubules, lysosomes, centrioles, lipofuscin, melanin, glycogen, lipid

Nissl substance is composed of rough endoplasmic reticulum and synthesizes protein. This is transported to the synaptic terminals along the axon via axoplasmic flow. The Nissl substance concentrates at the periphery of the cytoplasm following neuronal damage or fatigue and seems to disappear – this is known as chromatolysis.

Lipofuscin is a metabolic product which accumulates with age and is thought to be harmless.

Melanin is found in the cytoplasm of neurones in, for example, the substantia nigra and the locus ceruleus.

Neuroglia

Also known as interstitial cells, the neuroglia make up most of the nervous tissue, outnumbering neurones five to ten times.

Astrocytes (astroglia)

Some of their processes end as perivascular feet on capillaries. This gliovascular membrane helps form the blood–brain barrier.

There are two types of astrocytes:

• Fibrous
○ mainly in white matter
○ processes are relatively long and thin

- Protoplasmic
  - mainly in grey matter
  - processes are relatively short and thick

Oligodendrocytes (oligodendroglia)

Compared with astrocytes, oligodendrocytes have a smaller perikaryon, with fewer processes. Form myelin sheaths of CNS nerve fibres.

Microglia

The smallest neuroglial cells. CNS injury activates the microglia which then migrate to the site of injury. Here they are phagocytic and remove the debris.

Ependyma

Line the cavities of the CNS. Types:

- Ependymocytes – line the central canal of the spinal cord and the ventricles
- Tanycytes – line the third ventricle floor over the hypothalamic median eminence
- Choroidal epithelial cells – cover the surfaces of the choroidal plexuses and have tight junctions

Schwann cells

Form myelin sheaths of peripheral nerve axons. Encircle some unmyelinated peripheral nerve axons.

Segmental innervation of the skin

A dermatome is the skin area supplied by a spinal nerve. For neurological examination and diagnosis it is important to have a knowledge of the dermatomes. The following is a guide:

    C5 to T1 – upper limb
         C7 – ventral and dorsal aspects of the middle finger
        T10 – umbilical region
         L1 – inguinal region
    L2 to L3 – anterior aspect of the upper leg
    L4 to L5 – anterior aspect of the lower leg
         S1 – posterior aspect of the lower leg and lateral aspect of the foot and sole

Sectioning of one dorsal root will not cause clinically detectable sensory loss because there is considerable overlapping of adjacent dermatomes.

There is greater overlap of fibres for pain, heat and cold than for fibres for light touch. Therefore sectioning of spinal nerves will cause an area of tactile loss which is greater than the area of loss of sensations of pain, heat and cold.

Segmental innervation of muscles

Biceps brachii tendon reflex – C5–**6**
Triceps tendon reflex – C6–**7**, and **8**
Brachioradialis tendon reflex – C5–**6**, and 7
Patellar tendon reflex – L2, **3** and **4**
Achilles tendon reflex – S**1** and **2**

The spinal cord

Figure 1.2 shows the major ascending tracts of the spinal cord in diagrammatic form.

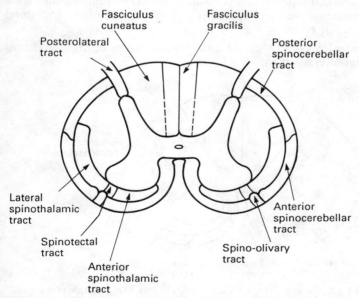

Figure 1.2 Diagram showing ascending tracts in a transverse section of the spinal cord

Ascending anterior white column tracts

- Anterior spinothalamic tract–light touch and pressure sense

Ascending lateral white column tracts

- Anterior spinocerebellar tract – proprioceptive, pressure and touch information
- Lateral spinothalamic tract – pain and temperature sense
- Posterior spinocerebellar tract – proprioceptive, pressure and touch information
- Spino-olivary tract – proprioceptive and cutaneous information
- Spinotectal tract – spinovisual reflexes

Ascending posterior white column tracts

- Fasciculus cuneatus and fasciculus gracilis – discriminative touch, proprioception, and vibration sense

Summary of major sensory pathways for information from general sensory endings to the thalamus and sensory cortex

- Light touch and pressure – contralateral anterior spinothalamic tract
- Pain and temperature – contralateral lateral spinothalamic tract
- Discriminative touch, proprioception and vibration – ipsilateral posterior column

Figure 1.3 shows the major descending tracts of the spinal cord in diagrammatic form.

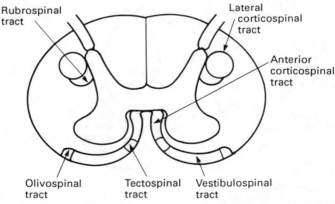

Figure 1.3 Diagram showing descending tracts in a transverse section of the spinal cord. Note that the exact location of the lateral reticulospinal tracts are not known for certain

Descending anterior white column tracts

- Anterior corticospinal tract – voluntary movement
- Reticulospinal fibres – motor function
- Tectospinal tract – part of a reflex for turning the head and moving the upper limbs in response to acoustic, cutaneous and visual stimuli
- Vestibulospinal tract – muscle tone control

Descending lateral white column tracts

- Lateral corticospinal tract – voluntary movement
- Rubrospinal tract – muscular activity
- Lateral reticulospinal tract – muscular activity
- Descending autonomic fibres – visceral function control
- Olivospinal tract – ? muscular activity

Developmental organization of the brain

At an early stage, the midline neural tube differentiates into the following vesicles (see Figure 1.4):

- The prosencephalon or forebrain, which later differentiates into
  - telencephalon
  - diencephalon
- The mesencephalon or midbrain
- The rhombencephalon or hindbrain, which later differentiates into
  - metencephalon
  - myelencephalon

Telencephalon

Gives rise to the cerebral hemispheres, including:

- The pallium or cerebral cortex
- The rhinencephalon or nosebrain, consisting of
  - the olfactory mucosa
  - the olfactory bulbs
  - the olfactory tracts
  - a strip of paleocortex from the temporal lobe uncus to the medial surface of the frontal lobe

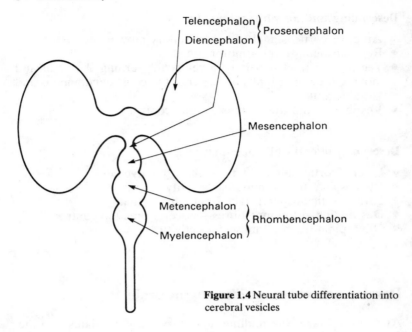

Figure 1.4 Neural tube differentiation into cerebral vesicles

- The corpus striatum, consisting of
  - the caudate nucleus
  - the lenticular nucleus, which is divided into:
    - the putamen
    - the globus pallidus
- The medullary centre, consisting of
  - fibres connecting cortical areas of the same cerebral hemisphere
  - fibres connecting cortical areas of both cerebral hemispheres by crossing the midline in the corpus callosum
  - fibres passing in both directions between the cerebral cortex and subcortical centres

Many textbooks use the term basal ganglia as being synonymous with the corpus striatum. Strictly speaking, however, the basal ganglia of the telencephalon consist of:

- The amygdaloid nucleus
- The claustrum
- The corpus striatum

Diencephalon

Consists of the following structures on each side:
- The thalamus
- The subthalamus
- The epithalamus, which comprises
  - the habenular nucleus
  - the pineal gland
- The hypothalamus

Mesencephalon

Consists of:
- The tectum, which consists of the corpora quadrigemina, comprised of
  - the superior colliculi
  - the inferior colliculi
- The basis pedunculi
- The substantia nigra
- The tegmentum, containing
  - the red nuclei
  - fibre tracts
  - grey matter surrounding the cerebral aqueduct

Metencephalon

Consists of:
- The pons
- The oral part of the medulla oblongata
- The cerebellum

Myelencephalon

- This is the caudal part of the medulla oblongata

Organization of the cerebral cortex

Neurones of the cerebral cortex
- Fusiform cells
- Horizontal cells of Cajal
- Cells of Martinotti

- Pyramidal cells, including Betz cells, which are giant pyramidal cells found in the motor prefrontal gyrus
- Stellate cells

Layers of the cerebral cortex

Developmentally the pallium consists of:

- Paleocortex or primary olfactory area – three cellular layers
- Archicortex or limbic formation – three cellular layers
- Neocortex
    - makes up about nine-tenths of the human pallium
    - consists of six cellular layers, as follows:
        - the molecular or plexiform layer, the most superficial layer
        - the external granular layer
        - the external pyramidal layer
        - the internal granular layer
        - the ganglionic or internal pyramidal layer
        - the multiform or polymorphic cell layer

Cortical areas (Figure 1.5)

Frontal lobe
The entire area anterior to the central sulcus and superior to the lateral fissure on the lateral surface. Important cortical areas are:

- The precentral area, which comprises:
    - a posterior region, the primary motor area
        - contains the giant pyramidal cells of Betz
        - concerned with voluntary movement
        - experimental electrical stimulation leads to contraction of muscle groups causing contralateral movements, e.g. in the limbs, or bilateral movements, e.g. in the upper face
        - movements are controlled by an area of cortex proportional to their complexity
    - an anterior region, the premotor or secondary motor area
        - no giant pyramidal cells of Betz
        - compared with the primary motor cortex stronger experimental electrical stimulation is required to cause the same degree of movement
- The supplementary motor cortex
    - compared with the primary motor cortex stronger experimental electrical stimulation is required to cause the same degree of movement

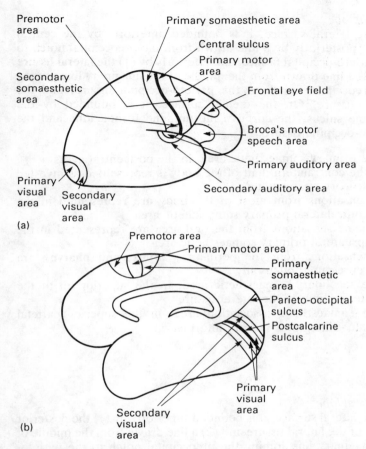

Figure 1.5 Localization of function in the cerebral cortex: (a) lateral aspect; (b) medial aspect

- The frontal eye field or eye motor field
  - experimental electrical stimulation leads to conjugate eye movements
- Broca's motor speech area
  - present in the dominant cerebral hemisphere
  - lesions affect the motor aspect of speech
- The prefrontal cortex, a large area lying anterior to the precentral area
  - concerned with personality, depth of feeling, initiative and judgement

Parietal lobe

On the lateral surface, it is bounded anteriorly by the central sulcus, posteriorly by a line drawn from the preoccipital notch to the parieto-occipital fissure, and inferiorly by (1) the lateral fissure and (2) a line drawn from the middle of the imaginary line joining the preoccipital notch to the parieto-occipital fissure, and the lateral fissure. On the medial surface, it is bounded by the calcarine sulcus, the corpus callosum, the frontal lobe and the parieto-occipital fissure.

- The primary somaesthetic area, in the postcentral gyrus
  - the contralateral half of the body is represented as inverted sensory homunculus
  - sensations from most of the body are represented in the contralateral primary somaesthetic area
  - some sensations from the oral area are represented in the ipsilateral primary somaesthetic area
  - sensations from the perineum, larynx, and pharynx are represented bilaterally
- The secondary somaesthetic area, in the superior lip of the posterior limb of the lateral fissure
- The somaesthetic association area, in the superior parietal lobule – integrates sensory information

Temporal lobe

On the lateral surface, it is bounded superiorly by (1) the posterior ramus of the lateral fissure and (2) a line drawn from the middle of the imaginary line joining the preoccipital notch to the parieto-occipital fissure, and the lateral fissure, and posteriorly by a line drawn from the preoccipital notch to the parieto-occipital fissure. The inferior surface is bounded posteriorly by a line drawn from the preoccipital notch to the anterior end of the calcarine sulcus.

- The primary auditory area, in the floor of the lateral fissure and extending slightly on the lateral cerebral hemisphere
  - its afferent fibres are from the medial geniculate body, forming the auditory radiation of the internal capsule
  - a unilateral lesion leads to partial loss of hearing in both ears
- The secondary auditory area, posterior to the primary auditory area
  - may be involved in the interpretation of sounds

Occipital lobe

On the lateral surface, it is bounded anteriorly by a line drawn from the preoccipital notch to the parieto-occipital fissure. On the medial surface it is separated from the temporal lobe as described above.

- The primary visual area, in the upper and lower lips of the calcarine sulcus on the medial surface of the cerebral hemisphere
  - its afferent fibres are from the lateral geniculate body of the ipsilateral thalamus
  - receives visual information from the contralateral field of vision, i.e. from the
    - ipsilateral temporal retina
    - contralateral nasal retina
  - the superior wall of the calcarine sulcus receives visual information from the contralateral inferior field of vision, i.e. from the superior retinal quadrants
  - the inferior wall of the calcarine sulcus receives visual information from the contralateral superior field of vision, i.e. from the inferior retinal quadrants
- The secondary visual area, which surrounds the primary visual area
  - its afferent fibres are from
    - the primary visual area
    - other cortical areas
    - the thalamus
  - may contain the occipital eye field; experimental electrical stimulation leads to conjugate eye movements

Insula

This area of cortex, also known as the island of Reil, lies at the bottom of the lateral fissure, and is hidden from view unless the lips of the lateral fissure are separated. It may be bound to the corpus striatum during fetal development, and its functions and connections are not fully known.

Cranial nerves

Olfactory nerve (I)

Olfactory receptor central processes pass from the olfactory mucosa, superiorly through the cribriform plate of the ethmoid bone, and synapse with the olfactory bulb mitral cells. From here the mitral cell axons pass in the olfactory tract, via the lateral olfactory striae, to the periamygdaloid and prepiriform areas of the cerebral cortex.

Optic nerve (II) and visual pathway

The optic nerve is formed by the axons of the retinal ganglion cells. In the optic chiasma, medial retinal fibres (carrying information from the temporal visual field) cross over to the contralateral optic tract. Lateral retinal fibres (carrying information from the nasal visual field) pass to the ipsilateral optic tract.

Most of the optic tract fibres synapse with neurones in the lateral geniculate body of the thalamus. A few optic tract fibres, concerned with pupillary and ocular reflexes, by-pass the lateral geniculate body and pass to the pretectal nucleus and the superior colliculi.

From the lateral geniculate body the fibres of the optic radiation pass to the visual cortex.

Oculomotor nerve (III)

This cranial nerve has two motor nuclei:

- The main oculomotor nucleus, which is in the grey matter surrounding the cerebral aqueduct of the midbrain, at the level of the superior colliculi – supplies all the extrinsic ocular muscles except the superior oblique and the the lateral rectus
- The accessory parasympathetic or Edinger–Westphal nucleus, which is posterior to the main oculomotor nucleus
  - preganglionic parasympathetic fibres pass to the ciliary ganglion
  - ciliary ganglion efferent fibres pass to the ciliary muscle and the constrictor pupillae of the iris, via about ten short ciliary nerves
  - stimulation leads to pupil constriction and lens accommodation

Trochlear nerve (IV)

The nucleus is in the grey matter surrounding the cerebral aqueduct of the midbrain, at the level of the inferior colliculi
  It supplies one ocular muscle, the superior oblique.

Trigeminal nerve (V)

This, the largest cranial nerve, has four nuclei:

- The main sensory nucleus, which is in the posterior pons
- The spinal nucleus, which is continuous with the above nucleus superiorly, and passes through the medulla inferiorly to C2
- The mesencephalic nucleus, which is in the grey matter surrounding the cerebral aqueduct, and passes inferiorly into the pons
- The motor nucleus, which is in the pons

Sensory components

The trigeminal nerve is the main sensory nerve to most of the head and face. There are three main divisions:

- The ophthalmic nerve or division
  - the frontal nerve supplies the upper eyelid and the scalp (anterior to the lambdoid suture), via the supratrochlear and supraorbital nerves
  - the lacrimal nerve supplies the lacrimal gland, the upper eyelid and the lateral conjunctiva
  - the nasociliary nerve supplies the eyeball, the medial lower eyelid and the nose (skin and mucosa)
  - sensory fibres end in the inferior part of the spinal nucleus
- The maxillary nerve or division
  - the infraorbital nerve supplies the skin of the cheek
  - the zygomatic nerve supplies the skin of the temple and cheek, via the zygomaticotemporal and zygomaticofacial nerves
  - the superior alveolar nerve supplies the upper teeth
  - supplies the sensory component of the sphenopalatine ganglion, whose branches include:
    - the nasal branches
    - the greater and lesser palatine nerves
    - the pharyngeal branch
    - the long and short sphenopalatine nerves
  - sensory fibres end in the middle part of the spinal nucleus
- The mandibular nerve or division
  - the buccal nerve supplies the mucous membrane of the cheek and part of the skin of the cheek
  - the auriculotemporal nerve supplies the skin of the temple and auricle

- o the lingual nerve supplies the anterior two-thirds of the tongue, and part of the mucous membrane of the mouth
- o the inferior alveolar nerve supplies the lower teeth, and the skin of the chin and lower lip
- o sensory fibres end in the superior part of the spinal nucleus

Motor components
The muscles of mastication, the anterior belly of the digastric, the mylohyoid, the tensor tympani and the tensor veli palatini are all supplied by the motor component of the trigeminal nerve.

Abducent nerve (VI)

The nucleus is in the upper pons, beneath the floor of the fourth ventricle.
It supplies one ocular muscle, the lateral rectus.

Facial nerve (VII)

This cranial nerve has three nuclei:

- The main motor nucleus, which is in the reticular formation in the lower pons
  - o supplies the muscles of facial expression, the auricular muscles, the posterior belly of the digastric, the stapedius and the stylohyoid
  - o corticonuclear fibres from the contralateral cerebral hemisphere are received by the part of this nucleus that supplies lower face muscles
  - o corticonuclear fibres from both cerebral hemispheres are received by the part of this nucleus that supplies upper face muscles
- The parasympathetic or lacrimal and superior salivary nuclei, which lie posterolateral to the above nucleus
  - o the lacrimal nucleus supplies the lacrimal gland
  - o the superior salivary nucleus supplies the nasal and palatine glands, and the sublingual and submandibular salivary glands
- The sensory nucleus, which is the superior part of the tractus solitarius nucleus, and lies near the main motor nucleus of the facial nerve – receives taste fibres, via the geniculate ganglion, from taste buds in the anterior two-thirds of the tongue, the floor of the mouth, and the hard and soft palates

Vestibulocochlear nerve (VIII)

This cranial nerve consists of two parts:

1. The cochlear nerve, which is concerned with hearing. Its fibres are the central processes of the spiral ganglion cells of the cochlea. They terminate in the posterior and anterior cochlear nuclei, which lie in the inferior cerebellar peduncle
2. The vestibular nerve, which is concerned with the maintenance of equilibrium. Its fibres are the central processes of neurones of the vestibular ganglion, which lies in the internal auditory meatus. They terminate in the lateral, medial, superior and inferior vestibular nuclei, which lie in the floor of the fourth ventricle.

Glossopharyngeal nerve (IX)

This cranial nerve has three nuclei:

- The main motor nucleus, which is in the reticular formation in the medulla oblongata, and is part of the superior part of the nucleus ambiguus
  - receives corticonuclear fibres from both cerebral hemispheres
  - supplies the stylopharyngeus muscle
- The parasympathetic or inferior salivary nucleus, which is inferior to the superior salivary nucleus and close to the superior tip of the nucleus ambiguus
  - receives inputs from the hypothalamus, olfactory system, tractus solitarius nucleus, and trigeminal sensory nucleus
  - preganglionic fibres from this nucleus enter the tympanic branch of the glossopharyngeal nerve and reach the otic ganglion via the tympanic plexus and the lesser petrosal nerve
  - postganglionic fibres supply the parotid gland via the auriculotemporal branch of the mandibular nerve
- The sensory nucleus, which is part of the tractus solitarius nucleus
  - receives taste information from the posterior one-third of the tongue

Vagus nerve (X)

This cranial nerve, which has the most extensive distribution of the cranial nerves, has three nuclei:

- The main motor nucleus, which is in the reticular formation in the medulla oblongata, and is formed by the nucleus ambiguus
  - receives corticonuclear fibres from both cerebral hemispheres
  - supplies the intrinsic muscles of the larynx and the constrictor muscles of the pharynx
- The parasympathetic or dorsal nucleus, which is in the floor of the fourth ventricle
  - receives inputs from the hypothalamus, the glossopharyngeal nerve, the heart, the lower respiratory tract and the gastrointestinal tract as far as the transverse colon
  - supplies the involuntary muscle of the heart, the lower respiratory tract, and the gastrointestinal tract as far as the distal one-third of the transverse colon
- The sensory nucleus, which is the inferior part of the tractus solitarius nucleus
  - receives taste information from neurones of the inferior ganglion of the vagus nerve

Accessory nerve (XI)

This cranial nerve consists of a small cranial root, and a larger spinal root:

- The cranial root supplies, via the vagus nerve, muscles of the soft palate, larynx and pharynx
- The spinal root is formed from fibres of neurones of the spinal nucleus, which lies in the anterior horn of C1 to C5; it supplies the sternocleidomastoid and trapezius muscles.

Hypoglossal nerve (XII)

The nucleus is in the floor of the fourth ventricle.

It supplies all the extrinsic and intrinsic muscles of the tongue, with the exception of the palatoglossus muscle.

Blood supply to the brain and spinal cord

The brain is supplied by the internal carotid and vertebral arteries, which lie in the subarachnoid space, and branches of which anastomose to form the circle or polygon of Willis, also known as the circulus arteriosus. The spinal cord is supplied by the posterior and anterior spinal arteries, together with the radicular arteries, which are branches of the deep cervical, intercostal and lumbar arteries.

Circulus arteriosus (Figure 1.6)

It surrounds the optic chiasma, and is formed by the following arteries:

- Anterior communicating artery
- Anterior cerebral arteries
- Middle cerebral arteries
- Posterior communicating arteries
- Posterior cerebral arteries

The anterior cerebral artery supplies the medial and superolateral aspect of the cerebral hemisphere, and parts of the lentiform and caudate nuclei and the internal capsule.

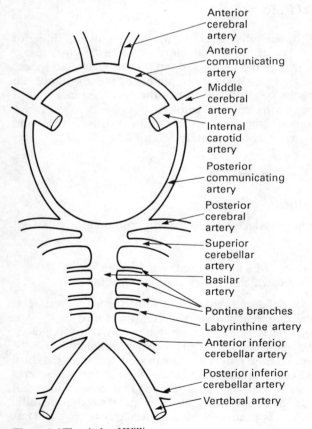

Figure 1.6 The circle of Willis

The middle cerebral artery supplies most of the lateral aspect of the cerebral cortex, the lentiform and caudate nuclei, and the internal capsule.

The posterior cerebral artery supplies the inferolateral aspect of the temporal lobe, the lateral and medial aspects of the occipital lobe, parts of the thalamus and lentiform nucleus, the medial geniculate bodies, the midbrain, the pineal gland, and the choroid plexuses of the lateral and third ventricles.

The anterior spinal artery supplies the anterior two-thirds of the spinal cord.

The posterior spinal artery supplies the posterior one-third of the spinal cord.

Cerebrospinal fluid

This is formed, by an active process, by the ependymal lining of the choroid plexuses of the lateral, third and fourth ventricles.

It circulates through the ventricles and the subarachnoid space. It is reabsorbed, by a passive process, mainly by the arachnoid villi of the dural venous system. The rest of the cerebrospinal fluid is absorbed by spinal villi and the lymphatic system.

The total volume of the cerebrospinal fluid in the ventricles and subarachnoid space is approximately 140 ml.

The ventricular system

Two lateral ventricles, each having

- An anterior horn, which is anterior to the interventricular foramen
- A body
- A posterior horn, which is in the occipital lobe
- An inferior horn, which reaches the temporal lobe

The cerebrospinal fluid enters the third ventricle from the lateral ventricles via the interventricular foramina (of Monro).

The third ventricle lies between the thalami, as a slit-like cleft. The floor of this ventricle is formed by the hypothalamus.

The cerebrospinal fluid enters the fourth ventricle from the third ventricle via the cerebral aqueduct (of Sylvius) in the midbrain.

The fourth ventricle lies anterior to the cerebellum and posterior to the pons and the superior part of the medulla oblongata. It is rhomboid shaped when viewed from above and has a tent-shaped roof.

The cerebrospinal fluid enters the subarachnoid space from the fourth ventricle via the median aperture (foramen of Magendie) and the lateral apertures (foramina of Luschka).

Specimen MCQ

The following is Question 23 taken from page 11 of the *Report to the Court of Electors, The Royal College of Psychiatrists Working Party for Review of the MRCPsych.* Responsibility for the answers is taken by the authors.

The posterior (dorsal) columns of the spinal cord convey sensory impulses concerned with:

A. Pain
B. Conscious proprioception
C. Light touch
D. Hot and cold sensation
E. Vibration sense

Answers

A. FALSE This is conveyed by the lateral spinothalamic tracts
B. TRUE
C. FALSE This is conveyed by the anterior spinothalamic tracts
D. FALSE This is conveyed by the lateral spinothalamic tracts
E. TRUE

Bibliography

De Groot, J. and Chusid, J.G. (1988) *Correlative Neuroanatomy,* 20th edition. Los Altos: Appleton and Lange.
Kaplan, H.I. and Sadock, B.J. (editors) (1989) *Comprehensive Textbook of Psychiatry,* 5th edition. Baltimore: Williams and Wilkins.
Kendell, R.E. and Zealley, A.K. (editors) (1988) *Companion to Psychiatric Studies,* 4th edition. Edinburgh: Churchill Livingstone.
Snell, R.S. (1987) *Clinical Neuroanatomy for Medical Students,* 2nd edition. Boston: Little, Brown and Company.
The Royal College of Psychiatrists (1985) *Report to the Court of Electors, The Royal College of Psychiatrists Working Party for Review of the MRCPsych.* London: The Royal College of Psychiatrists.
The Royal College of Psychiatrists (1987) *General Information and Regulations for the MRCPsych Examinations,* 8th revision. London: The Royal College of Psychiatrists.

Chapter 2

Neurophysiology

Syllabus requirements

In neurophysiology the candidate's knowledge of the physiology of the motor and sensory systems and the autonomic nervous system should be updated as the basis of neurological examination and diagnosis.

[The following neurophysiology topics are part of the MRCPsych Part II syllabus:

(a) The basic concepts in the physiology of receptors, neurones and synapses.
(b) General principles of the physiology of emotion, perception, sexual behaviour and aggression, and such factual aspects as have relevance to psychiatry.
(c) The development and localization of cerebral functions, and their relevance to the effects of injury to and disease of the brain.
(d) A basic understanding of the neuroendocrine system and its relevance to psychiatry.
(e) A basic knowledge of the physiology of arousal and sleep and an elementary understanding of the physiological basis of the EEG.]

The motor functions of the spinal cord and the spinal cord reflexes

Spinal cord organization

Anterior motoneurones
- Alpha motoneurones
  - give rise to large Aα fibres which innervate skeletal muscles
  - one fibre and the muscle fibres supplied by it constitute a motor unit
- Gamma motoneurones
  - give rise to large Aγ fibres which innervate the intrafusal fibres of muscle spindles

Interneurones
- o present throughout the spinal cord grey matter
- o interconnect with each other
- o interconnect with anterior motoneurones
- Renshaw cells
  - o small interneurones present in the anterior horn
  - o inhibitory cells
  - o transmit inhibitory signals to motoneurones, causing lateral inhibition

Sensory input to motoneurones and interneurones
- Monosynaptic pathway
  - o sensory fibres from muscle spindles
  - o terminate on anterior motoneurones
  - o forms part of the stretch reflex
  - o very rapid feedback allowed
- Polysynaptic pathway
  - o sensory fibres (other than from muscle spindles) terminate on interneurones
  - o signals can be modified
  - o forms part of complex reflexes

Propriospinal fibres
- o ascend and descend in the spinal cord
- o form part of the multisegmental reflexes

The muscle spindle

Innervation
- Type Ia fibre
  - o sensory
  - o innervates central part of the receptor portion of the muscle spindle
  - o high speed of transmission (approx. 100 m/s)
  - o forms the primary or annulospiral ending
- Type II fibre
  - o sensory
  - o innervates intrafusal fibres adjacent to the primary ending (on both sides)
  - o lower speed of transmission (approx. 40 m/s)
  - o forms the secondary ending
- Alpha motoneurone – see above
- Gamma motoneurone – see above

Stimulation
- When the whole muscle is lengthened, so too is the muscle spindle
- When the intrafusal muscle fibres contract with the extrafusal fibres staying the same length, then the central part of the receptor portion of intrafusal fibres is lengthened

Comparator function
- Excitation – when extrafusal fibre length is greater than intrafusal fibre length
- Inhibition – when intrafusal fibre length is greater than extrafusal fibre length

The stretch reflex

Also known as the muscle spindle reflex and the myotatic reflex.

- Neuronal circuit
  - type Ia fibre from muscle spindle enters dorsal root of spinal cord
  - synapses with anterior motoneurone in spinal cord
  - motor nerve fibre to muscle containing the same muscle spindle
- Dynamic reflex – reflex muscle contraction occurs following sudden stretch of the muscle
- Static reflex – reflex muscle contraction continues for up to several hours while the muscle is being stretched
- Negative reflex – dynamic and static inhibition occur when the muscle is suddenly shortened

Clinical aspects of the stretch reflex
Muscle jerks are used clinically to test the functional integrity of the stretch reflexes. When the muscle tendon is struck with a tendon hammer the corresponding muscle is stretched. This initiates a dynamic stretch reflex.

Segmental innervation of muscles
Biceps brachii tendon reflex – C5–6
Triceps tendon reflex – C6–7, and 8
Brachioradialis tendon reflex – C5–6, and 7
Patellar tendon reflex – L2, 3 and 4
Achilles tendon reflex – S1 and 2

Jaw jerk
- Analogous to limb tendon reflexes
- Brisk stretch of the masseter muscles
- Afferent pathway by cranial nerve V
- Efferent pathway by cranial nerve V

Hyperreflexia
This may have no pathological cause, and may simply be caused by the patient being anxious. It is therefore useful to confirm the presence of significant hyperreflexia, using

- The finger flexion jerk
- Hoffman's sign

Absent or diminished reflexes
The method of reinforcement should be used to confirm the presence of absent or diminished reflexes. Note that in rare cases all the limb tendon reflexes may be absent in patients who do not have a neurological cause. Note also that it is important to compare both the responses between the left and right sides of the same limbs, and the responses between the arms and legs.
   Causes of absent or diminished reflexes include:

- Muscle lesions
- Myoneural junction lesions
- Peripheral nerve lesions
- Spinal cord lesions

Reflexes may also be diminished by the patient being on regular hypnotic or anticonvulsant medication.

Clonus
This is said to be present when a sudden stretch of a muscle leads to a rhythmic series of involuntary contractions. Note that anxiety may be the cause of a few beats of clonus.
   Sustained clonus is caused by exaggerated tendon reflexes, owing to damage to the pyramidal pathway.

The tendon reflex

The Golgi tendon organ:
- Lies in the muscle tendon
- Connected in series with an average of 10–15 muscle fibres
- Detects muscle tension
- Transmits information via type Aα fibres to the spinal cord, and, via the spinocerebellar tracts, to the cerebellum

Functions
- Lengthening reaction – protective mechanism for the muscle and its tendons
- Servo mechanism for control of muscle tension

The flexor reflex

Also known as the nociceptive reflex and the withdrawal reflex. It refers to the reflex contraction of limb flexor muscles in the spinal or decerebrate animal following a sensory stimulus to the limb, classically a painful stimulus such as pinching or heat being applied.

Features
- Extrinsic reflex
- Comprises a spinal polysynaptic reflex arc
- It is protective

The crossed extensor reflex

Also known as the contralateral extensor reflex. It refers to the reflex extension of the contralateral limb approximately 0.2–0.5 second after a stimulus elicits a flexor reflex in a limb.

Painful stimulation of a limb activates the following motor reflex arcs at the segmental level:

- Excitation of the ipsilateral flexor motoneurones (flexor reflex)
- Excitation of the contralateral extensor motoneurones (crossed extensor reflex)
- Inhibition of the ipsilateral extensor motoneurones
- Inhibition of the contralateral flexor motoneurones

Reciprocal innervation

This refers to the phenomenon whereby excitation of one group of muscles may be associated with inhibition of a group of antagonistic muscles. It is illustrated above by the motor reflex arcs at the segmental level that are activated by painful stimulation of a limb.

Rebound
This refers to the phenomenon whereby, following a reflex, a second reflex of the same type as the first is more difficult to elicit during a given period of time. During this period of time reflexes of antagonistic muscles are easier to elicit, owing to reciprocal innervation.

Postural and locomotive reflexes of the spinal cord

The positive supportive reaction
This refers to the phenomenon whereby, following the application of pressure on the footpad of a decerebrate animal, the limb reflexly extends against the pressure.

The magnet reaction
This refers to the phenomenon whereby, in the positive supportive reaction the bottom of the foot remains extended towards the pressure, whatever the direction of application of that pressure.

The cord righting reflex
This refers to the phenomenon whereby a spinal animal will try to right itself to standing position after being placed on its side.

The stepping reflex
This refers to the phenomenon whereby a spinal animal may demonstrate rhythmic stepping movements in its limbs.

Reciprocal stepping reflex
This refers to the phenomenon whereby when the stepping reflex occurs in one limb, it also occurs, but in the opposite direction, in the contralateral limb. It is caused by reciprocal innervation and is abolished if the spinal cord is sectioned down the centre so that the two limbs are no longer neuronally connected.

Spinal shock

This refers to the phenomenon whereby, following sudden transection of the spinal cord all the functions of the spinal cord, including the spinal cord reflexes, essentially disappear. The spinal neurones gradually regain their normal functioning after a few days to a few months in many animals. However, this return may be delayed for much longer in humans, and sometimes it is not complete.
    Some of the functions affected in humans include:

- Abolition of the sacral reflexes involved in bladder and bowel evacuation – may last several weeks but usually return
- Immediate fall in the arterial blood pressure – may last a few days but usually returns to normal
- Abolition of skeletal muscle reflexes integrated in spinal cord
    ○ may take several months to return to normal
    ○ some reflexes may eventually become hyperexcitable

o reflexes return in the following order
  – stretch reflex
  – flexor reflexes
  – postural reflexes
  – parts of the stepping reflexes

Motor functions of the brain stem
The reticular formation

Sensory inputs
These include the following sources:

- Basal ganglia
- Cerebellum
- Cerebral cortex – particularly the motor cortex
- Hypothalamus
- Spinoreticular tracts
- Spinothalamic tract collaterals
- Vestibular tracts

Excitatory function
The bulboreticular facilitatory area, making up most of the reticular formation, is excitatory. Stimulation leads to an increase in muscle tone generally or in local areas.

Inhibitory function
The bulboreticular inhibitory area, consisting of a small part of the reticular formation in the inferior medulla, is inhibitory. Stimulation leads to a decrease in muscle tone generally or in local areas.

Antigravity support of body
Extensor muscle tone is maintained mainly by intrinsic excitation from the following:

- The bulboreticular facilitatory area
- The vestibular nuclei

The vestibular apparatus

Components
Bony labyrinth, containing the membranous labyrinth:

- Cochlear duct
- Three semicircular canals
- Utricle
- Saccule

Vestibular nerve
Its fibres are the central processes of neurones of the vestibular ganglion, which lies in the internal auditory meatus. They terminate in the lateral, medial, superior and inferior vestibular nuclei, which lie in the floor of the fourth ventricle.

Functions
The cochlear duct is involved with hearing.

The semicircular canals are important in the maintenance of equilibrium. Their particular functions include:

● The detection of angular acceleration
● The detection of angular velocity
● The prediction that malequilibrium is going to occur before it happens

The utricle and saccule are important in the maintenance of static equilibrium. In particular, the utricle is involved in the detection of linear acceleration.

Reflexes
The vestibular apparatus is involved in the following reflexes:

● The vestibular righting reflex
● The vestibular phasic postural reflexes

Stabilization of the eye gaze
When the head is moved, the semicircular canals send signals that allow the angle of gaze to change by an amount equal and opposite to the change in angle of the head. Reflexes are transmitted from the semicircular canals to the ocular nuclei via the following structures:

● The vestibular nuclei
● The cerebellum
● The medial longitudinal fasciculus

Nystagmus
Occurs when the semicircular canals are stimulated. There are two components, the fast and slow components.

Clinical tests of function
The following are tests for the integrity of vestibular apparatus functioning:

● Test for positional nystagmus
● Balancing test
● Barany chair test
● Ice water test

The basal ganglia

Components and functions of the basal ganglia

The corpus striatum consists of:

- Caudate nucleus
- Lenticular nucleus, which is divided into the
  - putamen
  - globus pallidus

As mentioned in Chapter 1, many textbooks use the term 'basal ganglia' as being synonymous with the corpus striatum. Strictly speaking, however, the basal ganglia of the telencephalon consist of:

- Amygdaloid nucleus
- Claustrum
- Corpus striatum

The following structures are closely associated with the basal ganglia system for motor control, and are considered by some textbooks to be part of the basal ganglia for this function:

- Red nucleus
- Substantia nigra
- Subthalamus
- Thalamus

The following structures, which are part of the basal ganglia proper, are believed not to be involved directly with motor function:

- Amygdaloid nucleus
- Claustrum

The basal ganglia form an important subcortical link between, on the one hand, the motor cortex and, on the other, the remainder of the cerebral cortex.

Motor functions of the cerebellum

Inputs to the cerebellum

Types of afferent fibre

- Climbing fibres – terminal fibres of the olivocerebellar tracts
- Mossy fibres – terminal fibres of all the other cerebellar afferent tracts

Afferents from the spinal cord

- Anterior spinocerebellar tract
- Cuneocerebellar tract
- Posterior spinocerebellar tract

Afferents from the vestibular nerve

- Directly through the ipsilateral inferior cerebellar peduncle
- Indirectly, via the vestibular nuclei, through the ipsilateral inferior cerebellar peduncle
- Afferents from the inner ear enter as mossy fibres and terminate in the flocculonodular lobe

Afferents from the cerebral cortex

- Cerebro-olivocerebellar pathway
- Cerebroreticulocerebellar pathway
- Corticopontocerebellar pathway

Other afferents

- From the red nucleus and the tectum

Intracerebellar nuclei

On each side, from lateral to medial, the four nuclei are:

- The dentate nucleus
- The emboliform nucleus
- The globose nucleus
- The fastigial nucleus

Outputs of the cerebellum

Efferent signals are sent to the following parts of the motor system:

- Basal ganglia
- Motor cortex
- Red nucleus
- Reticular formation
- Vestibular nuclei

Motor functions

The cerebellum receives information concerned with motor function, via the above pathways, as follows:

- Balance – from the vestibular nerve
- Involuntary movements – mainly from the inferior olive
- Sight – from the tectocerebellar tract
- Voluntary movements – form the cerebral cortex, muscle spindles, and tendon organs, via the pathways described above

The cerebellum may act as a comparator, coordinating precise movements by comparing the proprioceptive information from muscles with the motor cortex output.

Signs and symptoms of disease of the cerebellum

- Ataxia
- Disturbance of reflexes
- Dysarthria
- Dysdiadochokinesis
- Hypotonia
- Intention tremor
- Nystagmus
- Past pointing
- Rebound
- Postural changes and alteration of gait
- Vermis syndrome

Cortical control of motor function

The motor areas

Details of motor areas of the frontal cortex are given in Chapter 1 and are repeated here for ease of reference:

- The primary motor area
  - contains the giant pyramidal cells of Betz
  - concerned with voluntary movement
  - experimental electrical stimulation leads to contraction of muscle groups causing contralateral movements, e.g. in the limbs, or bilateral movements, e.g. in the upper face
  - movements are controlled by an area of cortex proportional to their complexity
- The premotor or secondary motor area
  - no giant pyramidal cells of Betz
  - compared with the primary motor cortex stronger experimental electrical stimulation is required to cause the same degree of movement

- The supplementary motor cortex – compared with the primary motor cortex stronger experimental electrical stimulation is required to cause the same degree of movement
- The frontal eye field or eye motor field – experimental electrical stimulation leads to conjugate eye movements
- Broca's motor speech area
  - present in the dominant cerebral hemisphere
  - lesions affect the motor aspect of speech

Afferents to the primary motor area

The following are some of the important sources of afferents:

- Subcortical fibres from other areas of the same cerebral cortex
- Subcortical fibres from the other cerbral cortex via the corpus callosum; thus the two primary motor cortices are connected
- Somatic sensory fibres from the ventrobasal complex of the thalamus
- Tracts from the basal ganglia and cerebellum via the lateral nuclei of the thalamus
- Fibres from other thalamic nuclei

Arrangement of the motor cortex cells

The cells of the motor cortex are arranged in columns, which in turn are arranged in six cellular layers, as follows:

- The molecular or plexiform layer, the most superficial layer
- The external granular layer
- The external pyramidal layer
- The internal granular layer
- The ganglionic or internal pyramidal layer
- The multiform or polymorphic cell layer

Each column appears to be involved in performing a specific motor function.

Stimulation of spinal cord motoneurones by the brain

Pyramidal tract

- Corticospinal tract
  - mainly terminates on interneurones in the dorsal horns of the spinal cord
  - a small proportion terminates directly on the anterior motoneurones
  - causes specific muscle contractions

Extrapyramidal tracts

- Reticulospinal tract
- Rubrospinal tract
- Tectospinal tract
- Vestibulospinal tract
  - ○ a large proportion terminates directly on the anterior motoneurones
  - ○ a small proportion terminates on inhibitory neurones which inhibit the anterior motoneurones
  - ○ cause less specific muscle contractions than the corticospinal tract
  - ○ cause general facilitation and inhibition, and gross postural signals

Others

The anterior motoneurones are also influenced by sensory information from the dorsal root sensory neurones and by the propriospinal tracts which carry information transmitted between segments of the spinal cord.

Physiology of the sensory systems

The physiology of receptors, neurones and synapses is covered in the syllabus for the MRCPsych Part II Examination, and therefore will not be dealt with in this chapter. Much of what is required for the MRCPsych Part I physiology syllabus has already been covered above; for example, the pathways of the dorsal columns and spinothalamic tracts has been partly covered in the chapter on neuroanatomy. In order to facilitate understanding and memory, some overlap has been allowed between what follows and Chapter 1.

Somatic sensory information

This enters the spinal cord via the dorsal or posterior roots. In the spinal cord, most large sensory nerve fibres, which are mainly type Aβ fibres, enter the posterior white columns, while smaller sensory nerve fibres, which are mainly type Aδ and type C fibres, synapse with neurones giving rise to the spinothalamic tracts. These smaller sensory fibres are joined by lateral collaterals from the larger fibres.

Segmental innervation of the skin

A dermatome is the skin area supplied by a spinal nerve. The following is a guide:

C5 to T1 – upper limb
      C7 – ventral and dorsal aspects of the middle finger
     T10 – umbilical region
      L1 – inguinal region
L2 to L3 – anterior aspect of the upper leg
L4 to L5 – anterior aspect of the lower leg
      S1 – posterior aspect of the lower leg and lateral aspect of the foot and sole

Sectioning of one dorsal root will not cause clinically detectable sensory loss because there is considerable overlapping of adjacent dermatomes.

There is greater overlap of fibres for pain, heat and cold than for fibres for light touch. Therefore sectioning of spinal nerves will cause an area of tactile loss which is greater than the area of loss of sensations of pain, heat and cold.

Summary of major sensory pathways for information from general sensory endings to the thalamus and sensory cortex:

- Light touch and pressure – contralateral anterior spinothalamic tract
- Pain and temperature – contralateral lateral spinothalamic tract
- Discriminative touch, proprioception and vibration – ipsilateral posterior column

Posterior white columns

Nerve fibres enter the posterior white columns in the spinal cord and pass rostrally to synapse with the cuneate and gracile nuclei in the medulla. From here the majority of medial lemnisci fibres decussate and pass to the thalamus, where each lemniscus terminates in the ventrobasal complex of nuclei. From here neurones project to the primary and secondary somaesthetic areas of the parietal lobe.

Anterior spinothalamic tracts

Fibres from dorsal horn neurones cross the spinal cord through the anterior commissure to enter the anterior spinothalamic tract. This terminates mainly in the thalamic ventrobasal complex of nuclei, as in the case of the posterior white columns. Collaterals from some of the fibres terminate in the bulbar and mesencephalic reticular areas.

Lateral spinothalamic tracts

Fibres from dorsal horn neurones cross the spinal cord through the anterior commissure to enter the lateral spinothalamic tract. This terminates mainly in the intralaminar nuclei of the thalamus. A few fibres, in particular the type Aδ fibres, terminate in the thalamic ventrobasal complex of nuclei.

Parietal sensory areas

- The primary somaesthetic area, in the postcentral gyrus of the parietal lobe
  - the contralateral half of the body is represented as inverted sensory homunculus
  - sensations from most of the body are represented in the contralateral primary somaesthetic area
  - some sensations from the oral area are represented in the ipsilateral primary somaesthetic area
  - sensations from the perineum, larynx, and pharynx are represented bilaterally
- The secondary somaesthetic area, in the superior lip of the posterior limb of the lateral fissure
- The somaesthetic association area, in the superior parietal lobule – integrates sensory information

The autonomic nervous system

Physiological anatomy of the sympathetic system

The preganglionic cell body lies in the intermediolateral horn of segments T1 to L2 of the spinal cord. It sends a fibre to the spinal nerve via the anterior root of the spinal cord. From here it passes, via the white ramus, to the sympathetic chain ganglion. The postganglionic nerve usually passes to the organ being innervated. Note that in the case of the adrenal or suprarenal medullae there is direct innervation by sympathetic preganglionic fibres.

Physiological anatomy of the parasympathetic system

- Approximately three-quarters of all the parasympathetic fibres are in the vagus. The parasympathetic or dorsal nucleus of the vagus, which is in the floor of the fourth ventricle:

- o receives inputs from the hypothalamus, the glossopharyngeal nerve, the heart, the lower respiratory tract and the gastrointestinal tract as far as the transverse colon
- o the vagus supplies the involuntary muscle of the heart, the lower respiratory tract, and the gastrointestinal tract as far as the distal one-third of the transverse colon
- The accessory parasympathetic or Edinger–Westphal nucleus of the oculomotor nerve:
  - o preganglionic parasympathetic fibres pass to the ciliary ganglion
  - o ciliary ganglion efferent fibres pass to the ciliary muscle and the constrictor pupillae of the iris, via about ten short ciliary nerves
  - o stimulation leads to pupil constriction and lens accommodation
- The parasympathetic or lacrimal and superior salivary nuclei of the facial nerve:
  - o the lacrimal nucleus supplies the lacrimal gland
  - o the superior salivary nucleus supplies the nasal and palatine glands, and the sublingual and submandibular salivary glands
- The parasympathetic or inferior salivary nucleus of the glossopharyngeal nerve:
  - o receives inputs from the hypothalamus, olfactory system, tractus solitarius nucleus and trigeminal sensory nucleus
  - o preganglionic fibres from this nucleus enter the tympanic branch of the glossopharyngeal nerve and reach the otic ganglion via the tympanic plexus and the lesser petrosal nerve
  - o postganglionic fibres supply the parotid gland via the auriculotemporal branch of the mandibular nerve
- The sacral parasympathetic fibres, from S2–3, and sometimes S1 and S4 also, form the nervi erigentes which supply:
  - o the external genitalia
  - o the lower ureters
  - o the bladder
  - o the rectum
  - o the descending colon

With the exception of some cranial nerves, the preganglionic parasympathetic fibres pass to the wall of the organ being innervated, where they synapse with postganglionic neurones.

Neurotransmitters

Cholinergic fibres
- Sympathetic preganglionic neurones

- Parasympathetic preganglionic neurones
- Only a few sympathetic postganglionic neurones, supplying
  - blood vessels in skeletal muscle involved in exercise and fainting
  - eccrine sweat glands of the skin

Noradrenergic fibres
- The majority of sympathetic postganglionic neurones

Autonomic effects

Eye
- Ciliary muscle: parasympathetic stimulation causes contraction
- Circular muscle of iris: parasympathetic stimulation causes contraction
- Radial muscle of iris: sympathetic stimulation causes contraction
- Smooth muscle of lids and nictitating membrane: sympathetic stimulation causes contraction

Glands
- Gastric
- Lacrimal
- Nasal
- Pancreatic
- Parotid
- Submaxillary

- Sympathetic stimulation causes vasoconstriction
- Parasympathetic stimulation causes secretion

Heart
- SA node (rate)
  - sympathetic stimulation causes stimulation
  - parasympathetic stimulation causes inhibition
- AV node and conducting tissue
  - sympathetic stimulation causes excitation
  - parasympathetic stimulation causes depression
- Muscle
  - sympathetic stimulation causes increased force of contraction
  - parasympathetic stimulation causes decreased force of atrial contraction
- Coronaries
  - sympathetic stimulation causes vasodilatation
  - parasympathetic stimulation causes constriction

Lung airways
- Smooth muscle
  - sympathetic stimulation causes relaxation
  - parasympathetic stimulation causes contraction
- Glands
  - Parasympathetic stimulation causes secretion

Gut
- Lumen
  - Sympathetic stimulation causes decreased peristalsis and tone
  - Parasympathetic stimulation causes increased peristalsis and tone
- Sphincters
  - sympathetic stimulation causes increased tone
  - parasympathetic stimulation causes decreased tone

Gallbladder and bile ducts
- Sympathetic stimulation causes inhibition
- Parasympathetic stimulation causes excitation

Liver
- Sympathetic stimulation causes release of glucose

Urinary bladder
- Detrusor
  - parasympathetic stimulation causes contraction
- Bladder neck and trigone
  - sympathetic stimulation causes contraction

Ureter
- Sympathetic stimulation causes inhibition
- Parasympathetic stimulation causes excitation

Kidney
- Sympathetic stimulation causes decreased output

Systemic blood vessels
- Abdominal
  - sympathetic stimulation causes constriction
- Muscle
  - sympathetic stimulation causes
    - constriction (noradrenergic)
    - dilatation (cholinergic)

- Skin
  o sympathetic stimulation causes
    - constriction (noradrenergic)
    - dilatation (cholinergic)
  o Parasympathetic stimulation causes dilatation

Penis
- Sympathetic stimulation causes ejaculation
- Parasympathetic stimulation causes erection

Skin
- Pilomotor muscle
  o sympathetic stimulation causes contraction
- Eccrine sweat glands
  o sympathetic stimulation causes secretion

Blood
- Coagulation
  o sympathetic stimulation causes increase
- Glucose
  o sympathetic stimulation causes increase

Basal metabolism
- Sympathetic stimulation causes increase

Adrenal cortical secretion
- Sympathetic stimulation causes increase

Mental activity
- Sympathetic stimulation causes increase

Adrenal medulla

Stimulation causes the release of relatively large quantities of the hormones adrenaline and noradrenaline into the bloodstream. This results in similar effects on the body as those of direct sympathetic stimulation, with the exception that these effects last much longer in the case of the blood-borne hormones.

Diseases involving the autonomic nervous system

Horner's syndrome
Caused by interruption of the sympathetic nerve supply to the orbit. Clinical features include unilateral:

- Anhidrosis
- Enophthalmos
- Miosis with normal reactions
- Partial ptosis

Argyll Robertson pupil
Usually caused by interruption of the fibres from the pretectal nucleus to the Edinger–Westphal nucleus by a syphilitic lesion. Clinically the pupil has the following features:

- Small and irregular
- No light reflex
- Constricts with accommodation

Frey's syndrome
Caused by postganglionic parasympathetic fibres of the auriculotemporal nerve joining the great auricular nerve during healing following injury to the parotid gland. Clinically, stimuli for salivary secretion cause the secretion of sweat in the skin of the face.

Specimen MCQ

Nystagmus is a recognized feature of:-

A. Menière's disease
B. Frey's syndrome
C. Phenytoin abuse
D. Horner's syndrome
E. Cerebellar lesions

Answers

A. TRUE This causes vestibular nystagmus
B. FALSE
C. TRUE Nystagmus is often seen in patients who have taken high doses of sedative drugs such as barbiturates and phenytoin
D. FALSE
E. TRUE

Bibliography

Bannister, R. (1985) *Brain's Clinical Neurology*, 6th edition. Oxford: Oxford University Press.
Bray, J.J., Cragg, P.A., MacKnight, A.D.C., Mills, R.G. and Taylor, D.W. (editors) (1986) *Lecture Notes on Human Physiology*. Oxford: Blackwell Scientific.
De Groot, J. and Chusid, J.G. (1988) *Correlative Neuroanatomy*, 20th edition. Los Altos: Appleton and Lange.
Emslie-Smith, D., Paterson, C.R., Scratcherd, T. and Read, N.W. (editors) (1988) *Textbook of Physiology*. Edinburgh: Churchill Livingstone.
Guyton, A.C. (1986) *Textbook of Medical Physiology*, 7th edition. Philadelphia: Saunders.
Kaplan, H.I. and Sadock, B.J. (editors) (1989) *Comprehensive Textbook of Psychiatry*, 5th edition. Baltimore: Williams and Wilkins.
Kendell, R.E. and Zealley, A.K. (editors) (1988) *Companion to Psychiatric Studies*, 4th edition. Edinburgh: Churchill Livingstone.
McGuffin, P., Shanks, M.F. and Hodgson, R.J. (1984) *The Scientific Principles of Psychopathology*. London: Grune and Stratton.
Plowman, P.N. (1987) *Neurology and Psychiatry*. Chichester: John Wiley and Sons.
Rubenstein, D. and Wayne, D. (1985) *Lecture Notes on Clinical Medicine*, 3rd edition. Oxford: Blackwell Scientific.
Schmidt, R.F.(1985) *Fundamentals of Neurophysiology*, 3rd edition. New York: Springer-Verlag.
Snell, R.S. (1987) *Clinical Neuroanatomy for Medical Students*, 2nd edition. Boston: Little, Brown and Company.
The Royal College of Psychiatrists (1985) *Report to the Court of Electors, The Royal College of Psychiatrists Working Party for Review of the MRCPsych.* London: The Royal College of Psychiatrists.
The Royal College of Psychiatrists (1987) *General Information and Regulations for the MRCPsych Examinations,* 8th revision. London: The Royal College of Psychiatrists.
Walton, J. (1985) *Brain's Diseases of the Nervous System*, 9th edition. Oxford: Oxford University Press.
Weller, M. (editor) (1983) *The Scientific Basis of Psychiatry*. London: Baillière Tindall.

Chapter 3
Neuropathology

Syllabus requirements

In neuropathology the candidate's knowledge of the principal neuropathological changes in degenerative disorders, cerebrovascular disorders and other conditions which may be referred to the psychiatrist should be updated as the basis of neurological examination and diagnosis.

Alzheimer's disease

The same pathological changes take place in both the senile and the presenile form of the condition.

Gross pathology

Brain
- Shrunken
- Sulci widened
- Ventricular enlargement

Histology

Light microscopy
- Cell loss usually most marked in the following layers of the cortex
  - the molecular or plexiform layer, the most superficial layer
  - the external granular layer
  - the external pyramidal layer
- Astrocytic proliferation
- Hippocampal granulovacuolar degeneration
- Increased fibrous gliosis
- Neurofibrillary tangles

- Neuritic plaques (formerly known as senile plaques)
- Shrinkage of dendritic branching

Electronmicroscopy
- Neuritic plaques
  - ○ amyloid core
  - ○ abnormal neurites surround the amyloid
  - ○ silver staining
  - ○ number correlate with degree of cognitive impairment
- Neurofibrillary tangles
  - ○ twisted filaments
  - ○ filaments are helically paired
  - ○ numbers correlate with degree of cognitive impairment

Biochemistry

Postmortem brain
- Reduced acetylcholinesterase activity
- Reduced choline acetyltransferase activity

Early onset
- Reduced dopamine-β-hydroxylase activity
- Reduced γ-aminobutyric acid (GABA)

Clinical features
- More common in women
- Usually presents with memory loss
- Apathy or labile mood
- Paranoid features may occur
- Progressive impairment of intellectual function
- Progressive deterioration of personality
- Parietal lobe dysfunction type features (see below)
- Parkinsonism
- Mirror sign
- Epilepsy
- The presenile form is more likely to lead to aspects of the Klüver–Bucy syndrome
  - ○ hyperorality
  - ○ hypersexuality
  - ○ hypermetamorphosis
  - ○ hyperphagia
  - ○ placidity

Pick's disease

Gross pathology

- Asymmetrical atrophy of
  - frontal lobes
  - temporal lobes
- Knife blade atrophy of the gyri

Histology

- Astrocytic proliferation
- Fibrous gliosis
- Neuronal loss most marked in the outer layers of the cortex
- Ballooned cells
  - swollen oval neurones
  - silver-staining inclusions (Pick bodies)

Clinical features

- More common in women with a peak age of onset between 50 and 60 years
- Personality deterioration with features of frontal lobe dysfunction (see below)
- Nominal aphasia
- Perseveration including the gramophone symptom
- Memory and neurological impairment

Huntington's disease (chorea)

Gross pathology

Atrophy of:

- Basal ganglia
- Cortex, particularly the frontal lobes

Histology

- Gliosis
- GABA neuronal loss most marked in the basal ganglia
- Neuronal loss most marked in the frontal lobes

Biochemistry

- Dopamine hypersensitivity
- Reduced GABA
- Reduced glutamic acid decarboxylase

Clinical features

- Autosomal dominant disorder that causes an insidious onset of choreiform movements and progressive global dementia
- Equal sex incidence with an average age of onset in the 30s
- Personality change
  - distractable
  - irritable
  - apathetic
  - low mood
- Ataxia
- Slurred speech
- Psychosis (especially paranoid)

Creutzfeld–Jacob disease

This condition is also known as Jakob–Creutzfeld disease. Subacute spongiform encephalopathy is a more severe variant.

Gross pathology

- Little or no gross atrophy of the cortex
- Ventricular dilatation common

Histology

- Astrocytic proliferation, particularly in the
  - basal ganglia
  - brain stem motor nuclei
  - cerbral cortex
  - spinal cord anterior horn cells
- Neuronal degeneration
- Spinal cord long descending tract degeneration
- Status spongiosus in the cortex

Clinical features

- A rare form of presenile dementia with an equal incidence in men and women
- Memory impairment and personality change
  - slowing
  - fatigue
  - low mood

- Parietal lobe dysfunction type features (see below)
- Seizures
- Myoclonic jerks
- Psychosis
- Extrapyramidal features
- Dysarthria
- Dysphagia

Punch drunk syndrome

Gross pathology

- Cerebral atrophy
- Perforation of the septum pellucidum may be present
- Regions particularly affected are the cerebral cortex and the hippocampal–limbic area

Histology

- Cortical neuronal loss
- Neurofibrillary degeneration

Clinical features

- Occurs in patients who have suffered repeated head injuries, for example professional boxers
- Cerebellar features
- Extrapyramidal features
- Pyramidal features
- Impairment of memory and intellect
- Deterioration of personality

Normal pressure hydrocephalus

Hydrocephalus, a diffuse enlargement of the ventricular system, can be divided into the following types:

- Obstructive hydrocephalus
  - a block exists to CSF circulation
  - usually non-communicating (the ventricles do not communicate freely with the subarachnoid space)
- Non-obstructive hydrocephalus
  - ventricular enlargement is secondary to cerebral atrophy
  - communicating

In normal pressure hydrocephalus the situation is different to the above types with the hydrocephalus being both obstructive and communicating. It is caused by a block in the subarachnoid space which prevents the CSF from being reabsorbed. The pressure in the ventricular system is often normal, so that features such as headache are usually absent.

Clinical features

- Predominantly affects patients in their 60s and 70s
- There may be a history of head injury, subarachnoid haemorrhage, or meningitis
- Memory impairment
- Physical and mental slowness
- Unsteady gait
- Urinary incontinence

Wernicke–Korsakoff syndrome

Wernicke's encephalopathy, which is caused by deficiency of thiamine (vitamin B_1), may develop into Korsakoff's psychosis.

Pathological changes in Wernicke's encephalopathy

Petechial haemorrhages in

- Mamillary bodies
- Periaqueductal grey matter
- The walls of the third ventricle
- The floor of the fourth ventricle
- Inferior colliculi

Clinical features of Wernicke's encephalopathy

- There may be a history of a condition that may lead to thiamine deficiency, for example
  - chronic alcoholism
  - lesions of the stomach, duodenum or jejunum (for example gastric carcinoma) causing malabsorption
  - hyperemesis
  - starvation
- Peripheral neuropathy
- Ataxia
- Ophthalmoplegia and nystagmus
- Clouding of consciousness

Pathological changes in Korsakoff's psychosis

- Parenchymal loss
- Petechial haemorrhages
- Proliferation of blood vessels

Clinical features of Korsakoff's psychosis

- There may be a history of:
  ○ conditions such as chronic alcoholism that may lead to thiamine deficiency (see above)
  ○ carbon monoxide poisoning
  ○ head injury
  ○ anaesthetic accidents
  ○ heavy metal poisoning
  ○ tumour
  ○ bilateral hippocampal damage (for example following neurosurgery)
- Disorientation
- Impaired recent memory
- Confabulation
- Lack of insight, and apathy or euphoria

Focal cerebral disorder: clinical features

The clinical features give an indication of the location of the pathology, but usually do not imply the nature of the pathology itself. For example, frontal lobe syndrome can be caused by a number of different disorders such as a tumour, trauma, Pick's disease and syphilis. The clinical picture seen in dysfunction of different areas is given below:

Frontal lobe

- Change of personality, with, for example
  ○ disinhibition
  ○ reduced social and ethical control
  ○ sexual indiscretions
  ○ financial and personal errors of judgement
  ○ elevated mood
  ○ lack of concern for the feelings of other people
  ○ irritability
- Impaired attention, concentration and initiative
- Aspontaneity, and slowed psychomotor activity

- If the motor cortex is affected (see Chapter 1) there may be
  - contralateral spastic paresis (seen earliest in the face usually)
  - grasp reflex
  - increased tendon reflexes
  - positive Babinski sign
  - gait decompensation
- Posterior dominant frontal lobe lesions may cause
  - apraxia of the face and tongue
  - primary motor aphasia
  - motor agraphia
- Orbital lesions may cause
  - anosmia
  - ipsilateral optic atrophy
- Motor jacksonian fits
- Incontinence, usually urinary

Temporal lobe

- Dominant temporal lobe lesions may cause
  - sensory aphasia
  - alexia
  - agraphia
- Posterior dominant temporal lobe lesions may cause features of the parietal lobe syndrome
- Non-dominant temporal lobe lesions may cause
  - hemisomatognosia
  - prosopagnosia
  - visuospatial difficulties
  - impaired retention and learning of non-verbal patterned stimuli such as music
- Bilateral medial temporal lobe lesions may cause amnesic syndromes
- Personality changes may occur which are similar to those caused by frontal lobe lesions
- Psychosis
- Epilepsy
- Contralateral homonymous upper quadrantic visual field defect

Parietal lobe

- Visuospatial difficulties such as
  - constructional apraxia
  - visuospatial agnosia
- Topographical disorientation

- Both visuospatial difficulties and topographical disorientation can occur with lesions of the dominant or non-dominant parietal lobe
- Dominant parietal lobe lesions may cause
  - primary motor aphasia (anterior lesions)
  - primary sensory aphasia (posterior lesions) which may include
    - agraphia
    - alexia
  - motor apraxia
  - Gerstmann's syndrome
    - dyscalculia
    - agraphia
    - finger agnosia
    - right–left disorientation
  - bilateral tactile agnosia
  - visual agnosia (parieto-occipital lesions)
- Non-dominant parietal lobe lesions may cause
  - anosognosia
  - hemisomatognosia
  - dressing apraxia
  - prosopagnosia
- Cortical sensory loss
  - agraphaesthesia
  - astereognosis
  - impaired two-point discrimination
  - sensory extinction
- Visual inattention
- Sensory jacksonian fits

Occipital lobe

- Dominant occipital lobe lesions may cause
  - alexia without agraphia
  - colour agnosia
  - visual object agnosia
- Simultanagnosia
- The following are more common with non-dominant lesions:
  - visuospatial agnosia
  - prosopagnosia
  - metamorphopsia
  - complex visual hallucinations
- Contralateral homonymous hemianopia
- Scotomata

- Cortical blindness may be caused by extensive bilateral lesions
- In cortical blindness the optic fundi appear normal and the pupillary light reflexes are present

Corpus callosum

- Acute severe intellectual impairment may occur
- Anterior tumours may cause frontal and parietal lobe dysfunction type features
- Diencephalic structure involvement may cause
  - akinesis
  - somnolence
  - stupor
  - postural abnormalities that may be similar to those seen in catatonic disorders
- If the communication between the dominant hemisphere speech centres and the non-dominant hemisphere is disrupted then the following may be seen in a patient in whom the left hemisphere is dominant
  - left-sided apraxia to verbal commands
  - astereognosis in the left hand

Diencephalon and brain stem

- Lesions in the region of the third ventricle, aqueduct, and posterior hypothalamus may cause
  - amnesia (of the Korsakoff type)
  - confabulation
- Lesions in the posterior diencephalon and upper midbrain may cause
  - hypersomnia
  - somnolence
  - akinetic mutism
- Intellectual impairment or occasionally a rapidly progressive dementia (for example with thalamic lesions)
- Frontal lobe dysfunction type personality change but with better preservation of insight
- Features of raised intracranial pressure (see below)
- Pressure on the optic chiasma from a lesion (such as a craniopharyngioma) may cause visual field defects
- Thalamic lesions may cause
  - parietal lobe dysfunction type sensory disorders
  - hypalgesia to painful stimuli

- Hypothalamic lesions may cause
  - polydipsia
  - polyuria
  - increased temperature
  - obesity
  - amenorrhoea or impotence
  - altered rate of sexual development in children
- Pituitary lesions may cause various endocrine disorders
- Brain-stem lesions may cause palsies of cranial nerves and disorders of long tract motor and sensory functions

Raised intracranial pressure

- Headache
  - throbbing
  - worsening by coughing and bending over
  - worse on waking
- Vomiting
- Rising blood pressure
- Falling pulse
- Papilloedema
- Changes in the level of consciousness
- Impaired cognitive functioning

Multi-infarct dementia

This condition is also known as arteriosclerotic dementia.

Gross pathology

- Arteriosclerosis of major arteries
- Atrophy is local or general
- Cerebral infarction
- Ventricular dilatation

Histology

- Multiple infarcted areas with the extent of this relating to the amount of cognitive impairment
- Multiple ischaemic areas
- Gliosis

Clinical features

- More common in men
- History and clinical features of hypertension usually present
- Acute onset
- Stepwise deterioration
- Focal neurological symptoms and signs
- Nocturnal confusion
- Fluctuating cognitive impairment
- Emotional incontinence and low mood

Cerebral arterial syndromes

Middle cerebral artery

- Contralateral hemiparesis
- Cortical sensory loss
- Contralateral hemianopia
- Aphasia (dominant hemisphere lesions)
- Agnosic syndromes and body image disturbances (non-dominant lesions)
- Clouding of consciousness

Anterior cerebral artery

- Contralateral hemiparesis (leg affected more severely than the arm)
- Grasp reflex
- Cortical sensory loss
- Motor aphasia
- Clouding of consciousness
- Personality change of the frontal lobe dysfunction type
- Changes in mental functioning similar to those seen in a global dementia
- Incontinence

Internal carotid artery

- May be asymptomatic if the circle of Willis is patent
- Otherwise may cause a middle cerebral infarction type picture
- Monocular blindness
- Unilateral loss of carotid pulse on examination
- Ipsilateral Horner's syndrome

Posterior cerebral artery

- Contralateral hemianopia
- Visual hallucinations
- Visual agnosia
- Spatial disorientation
- Visual perseveration
- Alexia without agraphia (if dominant occipital lobe and the splenium of the corpus callosum are affected)
- Contralateral thalamic syndrome
- Cerebellar ataxia
- Cortical blindness (bilateral infarction)

Vertebrobasilar system

The arterial branches in this system are shown in Figure 1.6. If the basilar artery is totally occluded this usually results in rapid death Partial occlusion of the basilar artery may cause

- Brain stem features
- Pyramidal features
- Ipsilateral cranial nerve palsies
- Ipsilateral cerebellar features

Owing to the distribution of this system a large number of other manifestations can occur following partial occlusions of the system, including, for example:
- Peduncular hallucinosis
- The locked-in syndrome
- States of bizarre disorientation
- Excessive dreaming

Neurosyphilis

Meningovascular syphilis

Pathology
- Endarteritis obliterans, leading to
  - arterial thrombosis
  - granuloma or gumma formation
- Hypertrophic pachymeningitis – thickening of cervical dura
- Meningeal exudate
- Meningitis
- Myelitis

Clinical features
- Headache (common presenting symptom)
- Lethargy, irritability and malaise
- Fibrosis of the meninges and endarteritis may cause cranial nerve palsy, especially of
  - II
  - III
  - IV
  - VIII
- Ischaemic necrosis may cause hemiplegia
- Meningeal posterior spinal root thickening may cause pain
- Meningeal anterior spinal root thickening may cause muscle wasting
- Delirium
- Dementia

Tabes dorsalis

Pathology
- Dorsal root sensory neuronal degeneration in
  - lower thoracic nerve roots
  - lumbar nerve roots
- Posterior white column atrophy

Clinical features
Dorsal root involvement leading to lightning pains
- Loss of propioception leading to ataxia (gait is wide based and stamping)
- Severe paroxysmal stabbing pains in the
  - abdomen
  - chest
  - limbs
- Paraesthesiae of legs
- Argyll Robertson pupils (see Chapter 2)

General paralysis of the insane

Also known as general paresis. Pathological changes include:
- Cortex
  - atrophy
  - neuronal degeneration
  - spirochaetes present
- Meninges
  - thickened
  - lymphocytic infiltration

Clinical features
- Impaired memory and concentration
- Frontal lobe dysfunction type changes in personality
- A depressive picture is seen in about one-quarter of cases
- A grandiose picture is seen in about one-tenth of cases
- Epilepsy occurs in about one-half of cases
- Manic elated, neurasthenic and schizophreniform pictures are also sometimes seen

Systemic lupus erythematosus

This condition is also known as disseminated lupus erythematosus and, when it involves the central nervous system, it can cause the following pathological changes in the cerebral cortex:

- Arteriolar inflammation
- Haemorrhage
- Microinfarction

Nervous system clinical manifestations include:

- Cranial nerve lesions
- Peripheral nerve lesions
- Depression
- Phobias
- Epilepsy

Disorientation and hallucinations may also occur, but when they do they are usually secondary to corticosteroid therapy.

Specimen MCQ

The following is Question 24 taken from page 11 of the *Report to the Court of Electors, The Royal College of Psychiatrists Working Party for Review of the MRCPsych*. Responsibility for the answers is taken by the authors.

Characteristic pathological features of senile dementia of the Alzheimer type include:

A. Selective atrophy of the frontal lobe
B. Neuritic plaques
C. Neurofibrillary tangles
D. Extensive atheroma of the cerebral arteries
E. Reduced acetylcholinesterase activity in the brain

Answers

A. FALSE There is gross generalized atrophy of the brain. Selective atrophy of the frontal lobes can occur in, for example, Pick's disease

B. TRUE

C. TRUE

D. FALSE This is not a characteristic pathological feature of senile dementia of the Alzheimer type, whereas it is a characteristic feature of multi-infarct dementia

E. TRUE There is also reduced activity of the enzyme choline acetyltransferase

Bibliography

Bannister, R. (1985) *Brain's Clinical Neurology,* 6th edition. Oxford: Oxford University Press.

De Groot, J. and Chusid, J.G. (1988) *Correlative Neuroanatomy,* 20th edition. Los Altos: Appleton and Lange.

Gelder, M., Gath, D. and Mayou, R. (1989) *Oxford Textbook of Psychiatry,* 2nd edition. Oxford: Oxford University Press.

Kaplan, H.I. and Sadock, B.J. (editors) (1989) *Comprehensive Textbook of Psychiatry,* 5th edition. Baltimore: Williams and Wilkins.

Kendell, R.E. and Zealley, A.K. (editors) (1988) *Companion to Psychiatric Studies,* 4th edition. Edinburgh: Churchill Livingstone.

Lindsay, K.W., Bone, I. and Callander, R. (1986) *Neurology and Neurosurgery Illustrated.* Edinburgh: Churchill Livingstone.

Lishman, W.A. (1987) *Organic Psychiatry: The Psychological Consequences of Cerebral Disorder, 2nd edition.* Oxford: Blackwell Scientific.

Macleod, J., Edwards, C. and Bouchier, I. (editors) (1987) *Davidson's Principles and Practice of Medicine* 15th edition. Edinburgh: Churchill Livingstone.

McGuffin, P., Shanks, M.F. and Hodgson, R.J. (1984) *The Scientific Principles of Psychopathology.* London: Grune and Stratton.

Plowman, P.N. (1987) *Neurology and Psychiatry.* Chichester: John Wiley and Sons.

Rubenstein, D. and Wayne, D. (1985) *Lecture Notes on Clinical Medicine,* 3rd edition. Oxford: Blackwell Scientific.

Snell, R.S. (1987) *Clinical Neuroanatomy for Medical Students,* 2nd edition. Boston: Little, Brown and Company.

The Royal College of Psychiatrists (1985) *Report to the Court of Electors, The Royal College of Psychiatrists Working Party for Review of the MRCPsych.* London: The Royal College of Psychiatrists.

The Royal College of Psychiatrists (1987) *General Information and Regulations for the MRCPsych Examinations,* 8th revision. London: The Royal College of Psychiatrists.

Trimble, M. (1981) *Neuropsychiatry.* Chichester: John Wiley and Sons.

Walton, J. (1985) *Brain's Diseases of the Nervous System,* 9th edition. Oxford: Oxford University Press.

Weller, M. (editor) (1983) *The Scientific Basis of Psychiatry.* London: Baillière Tindall.

Chapter 4

Neuropharmacokinetics

Syllabus requirements

Basic principles of pharmacokinetics should be revised in relation to the main groups of drugs used in psychiatry – anxiolytics, antidepressives, antipsychotics, sedatives/hypnotics, lithium and anticonvulsants. What is required is an understanding of the pharmacological principles relevant to the prescribing of drugs in psychiatry. The basic principles of drug action and interaction in relation to the above groups of drugs is dealt with in the next chapter.

Pharmacokinetics

This includes the following processes:

- Absorption
- Distribution
- Biotransformation
- Excretion

Absorption

Disintegration
- Depends on the pharmaceutical formulation
- For example enteric coating slows down the rate of disintegration

Solution
- Depends on the a number of factors, including:
  - particle size
  - the ambient pH
  - the pK_a of the drug
- the Henderson–Hasselbach equation is

$$pH = pK_a + \log_{10}([base]/[acid])$$

- Therefore it follows that a drug is 50% ionized when the pH is equal to the pK_a of the drug

From the alimentary tract
- The major absorption mechanisms are
  - active transport
  - diffusion (passive)
  - pore filtration
- factors which influence absorption include
  - gastric emptying
  - gastric pH
  - intestinal motility
  - food in the alimentary canal
  - intestinal microflora
  - area of absorption
  - blood flow

From the rectum
Advantages of this route over the oral route include:
- It overcomes the problem of patients who cannot swallow
- The stomach is by-passed and therefore so too are factors such as the gastric pH and gastric emptying
- First pass metabolism is reduced since the portal circulation is avoided to some extent

From intramuscular injection
- Lipid-soluble drugs are rapidly absorbed
- Low-molecular-weight, water-soluble (but lipid-insoluble) drugs are rapidly absorbed
- High-molecular-weight, lipid-insoluble drugs are slowly absorbed
- Irritant drugs that cannot be administered subcutaneously can often be administered intramuscularly
- Rate of absorption is increased following exercise since this increases muscle blood flow
- Conditions which reduce muscle blood flow lead to a reduction in the rate of absorption, e.g. in heart failure
- Used for depot injections, e.g. with fluphenazine decanoate (Modecate), a fatty ester is administered which slowly hydrolyses releasing the free drug
- In gluteal injections the outer upper quadrant is used in order to avoid sciatic nerve damage
- Certain drugs may cause sterile abscesses, e.g. paraldehyde
- Creatine phosphokinase is released, which may interfere with diagnostic cardiac enzyme assays

- This route is contraindicated in patients receiving anticoagulant treatment

From intravenous injection
- Advantages
  - ○ acts rapidly and therefore of use in emergencies
  - ○ dose can be titrated against the response of the patient
  - ○ large volumes can be administered slowly
  - ○ avoids first pass metabolism
- Disadvantages
  - ○ adverse reactions may occur rapidly
  - ○ rapid administration may lead to dangerously high blood levels
  - ○ it is difficult to recall the drug (compare stomach washouts with oral medication)
  - ○ risk of embolism of, for example, air
  - ○ risk of sepsis
  - ○ risk of thrombosis
  - ○ the drug may accidentally be injected into tissues surrounding a vein leading to, for example, necrosis
  - ○ the drug may accidentally be injected into an artery leading to, for example, spasm
  - ○ cannot be used with insoluble drugs

Others
Other sites of absorption are rarely or never used with psychotropic drugs, e.g. absorption through the skin and lungs, and subcutaneous and intraperitoneal injections. They are therefore not dealt with further in this book.

Distribution

This refers to the distribution of a given drug between the body lipid, protein and water components. Factors influencing the rate and degree of distribution include the following.

Haemodynamic factors
- The most highly perfused organs receive the highest concentrations of the drug soon after absorption
- There is gradual redistribution to tissues and organs with lower blood flow rates such as resting skeletal muscle and adipose tissue
- Reservoirs for drugs include plasma proteins, muscle and, especially in the obese, fat

Permeability factors
- The capillary endothelium is highly permeable except in the brain (see below)
- Highly lipid-soluble drugs enter cells rapidly
- Highly water-soluble drugs enter cells slowly if at all

Blood–brain barrier
- Some astrocytic processes end as perivascular feet on capillaries and this gliovascular membrane helps form the blood–brain barrier (see Chapter 1)
- High rate of penetration for non-polar highly soluble drugs, and inhalational anaesthetics
- Low or nil rate of penetration for highly polar, water-soluble drugs and quaternary ammonium salts
- The stronger an acidic (low pK_a) or basic (high pK_a) drug, the slower the rate of penetration, because of the higher degree of ionization

Placenta
- Drugs may be transferred from the maternal circulation to the fetal circulation across the placenta by the following mechanisms:
  - active transport
  - diffusion (passive)
  - pinocytosis
- All drugs should be avoided during the first trimester, if possible
- Drugs may cause teratogenesis during the first trimester, with the third to the eleventh week being the time of highest risk
- Drugs may affect growth and development during the last two trimesters
- Drugs may affect the newborn child if given during labour
- Psychotropic drugs which should be avoided or used with caution during pregnancy are mentioned later in this chapter

Biotransformation

Note that not all drugs undergo biotransformation prior to elimination from the body, e.g. lithium. Biotransformation:
- Occurs mainly in the liver
- Other sites of biotransformation include:
  - kidneys
  - suprarenal or adrenal cortex
  - gastrointestinal tract

- ○ lungs
- ○ placenta
- ○ skin
- ○ lymphocytes
- Non-synthetic reactions include:
  - ○ oxidation
  - ○ reduction
  - ○ hydrolysis
- Synthetic reactions include:
  - ○ conjugation

Excretion

Occurs mainly via the following:
- Kidneys
- Liver
- Lungs
- Saliva
- Sweat
- Sebum
- Milk

Kidneys
- The most important organs for excretion of drugs and drug metabolites
- Factors influencing renal clearance include:
  - ○ glomerular filtration rate
  - ○ plasma drug concentration
  - ○ molecular weight of drug
  - ○ passive tubular reabsorption
  - ○ active tubular reabsorption
  - ○ tubular secretion
  - ○ lipid solubility
  - ○ degree of ionization
  - ○ the pK_a of the drug

Pharmacokinetic terms and equations

Conceptual compartment

$V_d = D/C$

where V_d is the volume of distribution

D is the mass of drug in the body at given time

C is the plasma concentration of the drug at a given time

The volume of distribution, V_d:
- ○ is the size of the conceptual compartment for the drug
- ○ does not have an anatomical meaning
- ○ usually does not equal an anatomical volume
- ○ does not have a physiological meaning

First-order elimination (linear kinetics)

Rate of elimination is directly proportional to the plasma concentration of the drug at a given time:

$dC/dt = -kC$
where k is a constant

Therefore it follows by integration that

$C = C_0 e^{-kt}$
where C_0 is the value of C at time zero

Whence

$\ln C = \ln C_0 - kt$

The elimination half-life, $t_{1/2}$, is the time taken for a given value of C to fall to half C. It is constant in first-order elimination.

$t_{1/2} = \ln 2/k$
where $\ln 2 = 0.693$ to three decimal places

The elimination clearance, CL, is the rate of elimination divided by the value of C.

$CL = V_d \cdot \ln 2/t_{1/2}$
Thus
$t_{1/2} = V_d \cdot \ln 2/CL$

Zero-order elimination (saturation kinetics)

Rate of elimination is constant; $t_{1/2}$ increases with the value of D:

$-dC/dt = V_{max}C/(K_m + C)$
where V_{max} is the maximum rate of decay of C
K_m is the value of C when $-dC/dt$ is $V_{max}/2$
K_m is the Michaelis constant

Intravenous administration

At a steady state, when

Rate of elimination = rate of intravenous infusion and C has the value C_{ss}

we have:

$$C = C_{ss}(1 - e^{-kt})$$
where $k = \ln 2/t_{1/2}$

Multiple dosing

The value of $t_{1/2}$ alone determines the time needed to reach steady state.

The mean steady-state concentration, C_m, is given by

$$C_m = Dt_{1/2}F/(V_d T \cdot \ln 2)$$
where T is the dose interval
$\quad\quad\quad$ F is a bioavailability factor ($F < 1$ for oral administration)

Since $1/\ln 2 = 1.44$ to three significant figures, it follows that

$$C_m = 1.44 Dt_{1/2}F/(V_d T)$$

Benzodiazepines

Absorption

Oral
• Good absorption
• Antacids reduce the rate of absorption of chlordiazepoxide

Intramuscular
• Less rapid than oral administration
• Lower peak values of C produced compared to oral administration

Intravenous
• High peak values of C

Protein binding
• High e.g. 95% for diazepam

Biotransformation

Desmethyldiazepam has a central position in the metabolism of benzodiazepines. For example:

Chlordiazepoxide $\longrightarrow$ desmethylchlordiazepoxide $\longrightarrow$ demoxepam $\longrightarrow$ desmethyldiazepam

Clorazepate $\longrightarrow$ desmethyldiazepam

Diazepam $\longrightarrow$ desmethyldiazepam and temazepam

Prazepam $\longrightarrow$ desmethyldiazepam

The liver is the main site of benzodiazepine metabolism.

Desmethyldiazepam $\longrightarrow$ oxazepam

Excretion

- Desmethyldiazepam has a $t_{1/2}$ of 96 hours
- $t_{1/2}$ increases with age
- V_d for diazepam increases with age

β-adrenoceptor antagonists

Absorption

Oral
- Good absorption
- Peak C between 1 to 3 hours

Protein binding

- High for propranolol
- Low for most of the other β-adrenoceptor antagonists

Biotransformation

The degree of metabolism varies. For example:

- Almost totally metabolized
  - alprenolol
  - oxprenolol
  - propranolol
- 40–60% metabolism
  - pindolol
  - sotalol
- Almost zero metabolism
  - atenolol
  - nadolol
  - practolol

Some β-adrenoceptor antagonist metabolites also act as β-adrenoceptor antagonists. For example:

Propranolol $\longrightarrow$ 4-hydroxypropranolol

Excretion

- The $t_{1/2}$ of the β-adrenoceptor antagonists varies
- For example, propranolol has a $t_{1/2}$ of less than 4 hours, whilst nadolol has a $t_{1/2}$ of more than 16 hours
- Chronic administration $\longrightarrow$ reduced first-pass hepatic metabolism $\longrightarrow$ increased $t_{1/2}$.

Tricyclic antidepressants

Absorption

Oral
- Good absorption
- Lipid soluble
- Anticholinergic effect following absorption $\longrightarrow$ decreased gastric emptying $\longrightarrow$ delayed oral absorption

Protein binding

- High, e.g. 90% for clomipramine
- High protein binding and large V_d $\longrightarrow$ poor dialysability in overdoses

Biotransformation

Initially there is usually side chain demethylation $\longrightarrow$ monomethyl metabolites with antidepressant properties. For example:

Amitriptyline $\longrightarrow$ nortriptyline
Imipramine $\longrightarrow$ desipramine

Ring hydroxylation also occurs.

Excretion

- High first-pass hepatic metabolism, e.g. over 50% for imipramine
- Large V_d $\longrightarrow$ relatively low C
- Long $t_{1/2}$, allowing oral administration once per day (usually at night)

Mianserin

This is a piperazinoazepine tetracyclic antidepressant.

Absorption

Oral
- Good absorption
- Peak C between 2 and 3 hours

Protein binding

- High

Excretion

- $t_{1/2}$ varies between approximately 8 and 19 hours

Monoamine oxidase inhibitors

Absorption

Oral
- Mostly lipid soluble
- Good absorption

Biotransformation

Hydrazine monoamine oxidase inhibitors are metabolized partly via acetylation. Thus toxic levels may be reached in slow acetylators.

Excretion

After stopping therapy with this medication, the inhibition of monoamine oxidase usually continues even when it is not possible to detect any remaining amount of the drug in the body. Therefore the dietary and drug restrictions (see Chapter 5) should be continued for at least 2 weeks following discontinuation of monoamine oxidase inhibitor therapy.

Neuroleptics

Absorption

Oral
- Incomplete absorption of chlorpromazine (a phenothiazine) with a bioavailability of approximately 30%
- Good absorption of haloperidol (a butyrophenone) with a bioavailability of approximately 60%

Intramuscular depot
- The gastrointestinal and hepatic first-pass metabolism that oral neuroleptics are subjected to are by-passed and thus there is an increased bioavailability

Protein binding
- High for chlorpromazine: 90–95%

Biotransformation

Chlorpromazine
- Conjugation with
  - glucuronate
  - sulphate
- Demethylation, forming
  - nor_1-chlorpromazine
  - nor_2-chlorpromazine
- Hydroxylation, forming
  - 3-hydroxychlorpromazine
  - 7-hydroxychlorpromazine
- Oxidation, forming
  - N-oxides
  - sulphoxides
- Many of the metabolites are pharmacologically active, for example 7-hydroxychlorpromazine has a dopamine receptor-blocking effect which is approximately the same as that of chlorpromazine itself
- Autoinduction of hepatic and intestinal mucosal enzymes occurs

Haloperidol
- Hepatic oxidative dealkylation
- Metabolites are thought not to be pharmacologically active
- Autoinduction of hepatic and intestinal mucosal enzymes has not been demonstrated

Excretion
- Chlorpromazine has a $t_{1/2}$ of between 2 and 24 hours; its high lipid solubility $\longrightarrow$ high V_d $\longrightarrow$ relatively low C
- Haloperidol has a $t_{1/2}$ of between 12 and 38 hours

Lithium

Absorption

Oral
- Lithium carbonate shows good absorption
- Peak C between 3 and 5 hours
- Controlled release preparations available, e.g. Priadel

Protein binding

- Nil

Biotransformation

- Nil

Excretion

- The $t_{1/2}$ increases with age, from approximately 18 hours in young adults to as high as 36 hours in the elderly
- Passes readily into the glomerular filtrate
- Reabsorption:
    - 70–80% proximal tubular reabsorption
    - zero distal tubular reabsorption
    - not affected by diuretics that act only on the distal tubule

Lithium and sodium cations compete for proximal tubular reabsorption. Therefore lithium retention can be caused by sodium deficiency and by sodium diuresis. Further details of the causes, effects and treatment of lithium toxicity appear in Chapter 5.

Carbamazepine

Absorption

Oral
- Generally slow
- Good absorption
- May affect gastric motility

Protein binding

- 75% at therapeutic concentrations

Biotransformation

One clinically important product which is itself antiepileptic is carbamazepine-10,11-epoxide.

Autoinduction of enzymes probably occurs.

Excretion

- Single dose: $t_{1/2}$ is approximately 25–60 hours.
- Chronic adminstration: $t_{1/2}$ decreases to 10 hours; this is probably caused by autoinduction of enzymes; therefore this drug needs to be taken approximately 12 hourly (twice daily)

Ethosuximide

Absorption

Oral
- Good

Protein binding

- Very low

Biotransformation

Two major pharmacologically inactive metabolites are formed by hepatic metabolism.

Excretion

- Children: $t_{1/2}$ is approximately 30 hours
- Adults: $t_{1/2}$ is approximately 70 hours
- Can be administered once daily

Phenobarbitone

Absorption

Oral
- Good
- Peak C may occur only after 6 hours

Intramuscular
- Good
- Peak C may occur only after 6 hours

Protein binding

- 50% at therapeutic concentrations

Biotransformation

Approximately half is metabolized to pharmacologically inactive products, mainly by hepatic parahydroxylation.

Excretion

The amount excreted unchanged in the urine varies from approximately 10 to 40%. It is an acidic drug ($pK_a = 7.4$) and the urinary excretion depends on the pH of the urine, as well as its volume. Forced alkaline diuresis is used in cases of poisoning.

- Children: $t_{1/2}$ is approximately 40 hours
- Adults: $t_{1/2}$ is approximately 100 hours
- Can be administered once daily

Phenytoin

Absorption

Note that the bioavailability is reduced if Ca^{2+} is administered with the phenytoin.

Oral
- Generally good but great individual variation
- Peak C at approximately 2 hours

Intramuscular
- Crystallizes out at injection site
- Slower absorption than orally
- Lower peak C than orally

Protein binding

- 90% at therapeutic concentrations
- Phenytoin is displaced from plasma protein binding by a number of other drugs (see Chapter 5).

Biotransformation

Mainly by hepatic parahydroxylation:

Phenytoin $\longrightarrow$ 5-parahydroxyphenyl-5-phenylhydantoin

Saturation of this enzymatic reaction takes place at phenytoin concentrations that lie within the therapeutic range.

Excretion

- Less than 5% is excreted unchanged
- $t_{1/2}$ is generally between 12 and 120 hours, but it is not possible to calculate a single $t_{1/2}$ owing to the occurrence of zero-order kinetics (see above).

Specimen MCQ

The pharmacokinetics of a drug X are known to be first order. The following statements are true:

A. The amount of X excreted unchanged in the urine is proportional to the dose of X
B. The half-life increases with the dose of X
C. The half-life increases with the plasma concentration of X
D. The steady state plasma concentration of X is proportional to the dose of X
E. First-order kinetics are also known as saturation kinetics

Answers

    A. TRUE
    B. FALSE $t_{1/2}$ is constant
    C. FALSE $t_{1/2}$ is constant
    D. TRUE
    E. FALSE Saturation kinetics are zero-order kinetics; first-order kinetics are also known as linear kinetics

Bibliography

Berrios, G.E. and Dowson, J.H. (editors) (1983) *Treatment and Management in Adult Psychiatry.* London: Baillière Tindall.
British Medical Association and The Pharmaceutical Press (1989) *British National Formulary,* No. 17. British Medical Association and The Pharmaceutical Press, London.
Crammer, J.L., Barraclough, B. and Heine, B. (1978) *The Use of Drugs in Psychiatry.* London: Gaskell.

Gelder, M., Gath, D. and Mayou, R. (1989) *Oxford Textbook of Psychiatry*, 2nd edition. Oxford: Oxford University Press.

Kaplan, H.I. and Sadock, B.J. (editors) (1989) *Comprehensive Textbook of Psychiatry*, 5th edition. Baltimore: Williams and Wilkins.

Kendell, R.E. and Zealley, A.K. (editors) (1988) *Companion to Psychiatric Studies*, 4th edition. Edinburgh: Churchill Livingstone.

McGuffin, P., Shanks, M.F. and Hodgson, R.J. (1984) *The Scientific Principles of Psychopathology*. London: Grune and Stratton.

Rogers, H.J. and Spector, R.G. (1984) *Aids to Clinical Pharmacology and Therapeutics*. Edinburgh: Churchill Livingstone.

Silverstone, T. and Turner, P. (1978) *Drug Treatment in Psychiatry*. London: Routledge and Kegan Paul.

The Royal College of Psychiatrists (1985) *Report to the Court of Electors, The Royal College of Psychiatrists Working Party for Review of the MRCPsych*. London: The Royal College of Psychiatrists.

The Royal College of Psychiatrists (1987) *General Information and Regulations for the MRCPsych Examinations*, 8th revision. London: The Royal College of Psychiatrists.

Tyrer, P. (editor) (1982) *Drugs in Psychiatric Practice*. London: Butterworths.

Chapter 5

Drug actions and interactions

Syllabus requirements

Basic principles of drug action and interaction should be revised in relation to the main groups of drugs used in psychiatry – anxiolytics, antidepressives, antipsychotics, sedatives/hypnotics, lithium and anticonvulsants. What is required is an understanding of the pharmacological principles relevant to the prescribing of drugs in psychiatry. (The methodology of clinical trials will be examined in the MRCPsych Part II, and is therefore not considered in this chapter.)

For each class of drug, the principal indications, contraindications, side-effects, and interactions with other drugs are given below. Note that only those principal indications relevant to psychiatry are mentioned.

Benzodiazepines

Indications

- Acute ethanol withdrawal
- Epilepsy
- Short-term relief of anxiety and phobic panic attacks
- Short-term relief of insomnia

As anxiolytics, benzodiazepines should be used only in cases of severe anxiety, and indeed many psychiatrists now only rarely use this class of drug owing to the side-effects (see below), particularly the development of tolerance.

Types

- Alprazolam
- Bromazepam
- Chlordiazepoxide
- Clobazam

- Clorazepate
- Diazepam
- Ketazolam
- Lorazepam
- Medazepam
- Oxazepam
- Prazepam

Contraindications
- Acute pulmonary insufficiency
- Respiratory depression

Side-effects
Anxiety
- Probably a rebound effect particularly with benzodiazepines with short half-lives

Confusion and ataxia especially in the elderly
- The elderly are more sensitive to the effects of this class of drugs, partly because of reduced elimination and increased tissue sensitivity
- Benzodiazepine-induced drowsiness increases with age
- Benzodiazepines commonly cause ataxia, confusion and falls in regular elderly users

Drowsiness
- After taking a benzodiazepine at night, for example for insomnia, drowsiness and lightheadedness may occur the following day

Physical dependence
- Withdrawal symptoms include
  o anxiety symptoms
    – anorexia
    – anxiety
    – dysphoria
    – fatigue
    – headache
    – muscular pains
    – nausea
    – shaking
    – sleep disturbance
    – sweating
    – tremor

  – visual disturbance
  – weight loss
 o distorted perception
  – illusions
  – paranoid ideation
  – psychosis
 o neurological disturbances
  – ataxia
  – epileptiform seizure

Psychological impairment
● With long-term use

Other side-effects which occur occasionally include:

● Changes in libido
● Changes in salivation
● Hypotension
● Rashes
● Urinary retention

Reported side-effects for which there is conflicting evidence:

● Aggression
● Cerebral atrophy

Interactions with other drugs

The effects on benzodiazepines are given:

● Antidepressants – potentiation
● Antihistamines – potentiation
● Cimetidine – increased plasma concentration
● Disulfiram
  o decreased hepatic metabolism leads to potentiation
  o especially with chlordiazepoxide and diazepam
● Ethanol – potentiation
● Opioid analgesics – potentiation
● Phenothiazines – potentiation

β-adrenoceptor antagonists

Indications

Anxiety
● Best for those with palpitations, tachycardia and tremor, not
  responding to benzodiazepines

DaCosta's syndrome

- This condition has some 20 synonyms, including:
  - cardiac neurosis
  - effort syndrome
  - hyperdynamic β-adrenergic circulatory state
  - hyperkinetic heart syndrome
  - neurocirculatory asthenia
- It is commonly considered as a clinical variant of anxiety disorder

Migraine prophylaxis

Types

- Acebutolol
- Atenolol
- Betaxolol
- Labetolol
- Metoprolol
- Nadolol
- Oxprenolol
- Penbutolol
- Pindolol
- Practolol
- Propranolol
- Sotalol
- Timolol

Note that some of the above β-adrenoceptor antagonists tend not to be used for the psychiatric indications given above; for example the only main indication for betaxolol hydrochloride is hypertension.

Contraindications

- Asthma
- Following prolonged fasting – for example in anorexia nervosa
- Heart block
  - second degree
  - third degree
- Heart failure
- Metabolic acidosis
  - for example in diabetes mellitus
  - β-adrenoceptor antagonists block gluconeogenesis

Side-effects

Cardiac
- Bradycardia
- Heart failure

Central nervous system
- Fatigue
- Hallucinations
- Migraine
- Nightmares

In diabetes mellitus
- Hypoglycaemia (β-adrenoceptor antagonists block gluconeogenesis)

Peripheral vascular
- Exacerbation of Raynaud's phenomenon
- Intermittent claudication
- Peripheral vasoconstriction

Respiratory
- Bronchospasm

Sexual
- Erectile dysfunction

Interactions with other drugs

- Adrenaline – severe hypertension
- Cardiac effects occur with the following drugs
    - diltiazem
    - diuretics with sotalol
    - lignocaine
    - nifedipine
    - prenylamine
- Cimetidine – propranolol interacts with cimetidine leading to increased concentration of propranolol
- Ergotamine – increased peripheral vasoconstriction
- Rifampicin – propranolol interacts with rifampicin leading to decreased concentration of propranolol
- Sympathomimetic amines – severe hypertension reported

Tricyclic antidepressants

Indications

- Depressive illness
- Nocturnal enuresis in children
  - amitriptyline
  - imipramine
  - nortriptyline
- Obsessional neurosis – there is no justification for clomipramine (a homologue of chlorpromazine) to be used preferentially in this condition
- Phobic disorder

Types

- Dibenzocycloheptanes
  - amitriptyline
  - butriptyline
  - nortriptyline
  - protriptyline
- Iminodibenzyls
  - clomipramine
  - desipramine
  - imipramine
  - trimipramine
- Other tricyclic antidepressants
  - dothiepin (thio analogue of amitriptyline)
  - doxepin (tricyclic dibenzoxapine)
  - iprindole (indole nucleus and cyclo-octane ring present)
  - lofepramine (tricyclic dibenzazepine)

Contraindications

- Heart block
- Hypomania and mania
- Recent myocardial infarction

- Interactions also occur with the following conditions (hence caution is required):
  - cardiac pathology (with heart block and recent myocardial infarction being contraindications, as above)
  - diabetes mellitus
  - epilepsy
  - glaucoma

○ hepatic impairment
○ hypertension
○ impaired renal function
○ pregnancy
○ prostatism
○ schizophrenia
○ thyroid disease

Side-effects

Autonomic (anticholinergic)
- Blurred vision
- Constipation
- Dry mouth
- Nausea
- Paralytic ileus (rare)
- Postural hypotension
- Sweating
- Tachycardia
- Urinary retention
- Vomiting
- Worsening of angle-closure (narrow angle) glaucoma

Cardiac
- Therapeutic doses
  ○ electocardiographic changes
    – flattening of T waves
    – prolongation of QT interval
    – ST depression
  ○ others (see under Side-effects, Autonomic above)
- Higher doses
  ○ atrial fibrillation
  ○ atrioventricular block
  ○ intraventricular block
  ○ ventricular flutter

Central nervous system
- Ataxia
- Behavioural disturbances (particularly in children)
- Confusion (particularly in the elderly)
- Convulsions
- Decreased rapid eye movement sleep
- Electroencephalographic changes
- Fine tremor

- Headache
- Hypomania
- Paraesthesiae
- Sedation (not with all tricyclic antidepressants)

Other uncommon central nervous system side-effects include:

- Agitation
- Aggressive behaviour
- Buccofaciolingual movements
- Choreoathetoid movements
- Delirium
- Dysarthria
- Myoclonus
- Nystagmus
- Peripheral neuropathy
- Tinnitus

Haematological (uncommon)
- Agranulocytosis
- Eosinophilia
- Leucopenia
- Thrombocytopenia

Hypersensitivity reactions
- Allergic cholestatic jaundice
- Dermatological reactions

Sexual
- Erectile dysfunction
- Impairment of ejaculation
- Orgasmic delay

Others
- Blood sugar changes
- Hepatic necrosis
- Oedema
- Raised alkaline phosphatase
- Raised hepatic transaminases
- Reduced serum cholesterol
- Weight gain

Withdrawal syndrome
Lasts for 1–2 days following sudden termination of medication:

- Akathisia
- Anxiety
- Headache
- Insomnia
- Malaise
- Nausea
- Sweating
- Vomiting

Interactions with other drugs

Unless otherwise stated, the effect on tricyclic antidepressants is given.

- Adrenaline and noradrenaline – potentiation of the pressor effects of adrenaline and noradrenaline may lead to hypertension
- Antihypertensive agents – antagonism of the antihypertensive actions of bethanidine, clonidine, debrisoquine, guanethidine and reserpine
- Antiepileptic medication – reduced tricyclic antidepressant plasma level
- Barbiturates – increased metabolism of tricyclic antidepressants leading to reduced plasma level
- Cimetidine – increased plasma concentration of amitriptyline, desipramine, doxepin, imipramine and nortriptyline
- Coumarin derivatives – anticoagulant action of coumarin derivatives potentiated
- Dexamphetamine and other amphetamine derivatives – cardiac arrhythmias, excitement, hyperpyrexia, hypertension
- Disulfiram – increased tricyclic antidepressant plasma level
- Ethanol – potentiation of sedative action
- Lithium – there may be a summation of the side-effect of tremor from both drugs
- Methylphenidate – increased tricyclic antidepressant plasma level
- Monoamine oxidase inhibitors
  - central nervous system excitation, hypertensive crisis, hyperpyrexia, coma
  - at least 14 days should elapse between stopping a monoamine oxidase inhibitor and commencing a tricyclic antidepressant

- Oral contraceptives
  - reduced effect
  - higher plasma levels leading to increased side-effects
- Phenothiazines
  - higher plasma levels leading to increased side-effects
  - potentiation of phenothiazines also occurs

L-Tryptophan

Indications

- Depressive illness

Contraindications

- No absolute contraindications are reported
- Caution is required in the following conditions:
  - bladder disease
  - disorders of tryptophan metabolism

Side-effects
Central nervous system
- Drowsiness
- Headache
- Nausea

Interactions with other drugs

- Monoamine oxidase inhibitors – central nervous system excitation, confusional states

Tetracyclic antidepressants
Indications

- Depressive illness

Types

- Maprotiline
- Mianserin

Contraindications

Similar precautions need to be taken as with tricyclic antidepressants, apart from the fact that the tetracylic antidepressants are less cardiotoxic.

Both maprotiline and mianserin are contraindicated in the following conditions:

- Hypomania and mania
- Severe hepatic disease

In addition, maprotiline is also contraindicated in the following conditions:

- Epilepsy
- Angle-closure glaucoma
- Recent myocardial infarction
- Severe renal disease
- Urinary retention

Side-effects

Similar to the tricyclic antidepressants, with tetracyclic antidepressants showing the following differences:

- Less cardiotoxic
- Less anticholinergic effects
- Grand mal seizures may occur at high dosage with maprotiline
- Agranulocytosis, arthritis, arthralgia, influenza-like symptoms and jaundice may occur with mianserin
- Patients being treated with mianserin should have a regular full blood count (every 4 weeks in the first 12 weeks)

Interactions with other drugs

- Antihypertensive agents – maprotiline may lead to antagonism of the antihypertensive actions of bethanidine, clonidine, debrisoquine and guanethidine
- Barbiturates – decreased maprotiline plasma level
- Ethanol – maprotiline and mianserin may potentiate the effects of ethanol
- Methylphenidate – increased maprotiline plasma level
- Monoamine oxidase inhibitors – at least 14 days should elapse between stopping a monoamine oxidase inhibitor and commencing a tetracyclic antidepressant
- Neuroleptics – increased maprotiline plasma level

Fluvoxamine

Indications

- Depressive illness

Contraindications

No absolute contraindications have been reported. Treatment of patients with hepatic or renal disease should begin at low dosage with careful monitoring.

Side-effects

- Nausea is the most common side-effect

Other side-effects include:

- Agitation
- Anorexia
- Bradycardia
- Constipation
- Drowsiness
- Tremor

Interactions with other drugs

- Monoamine oxidase inhibitors – at least 14 days should elapse between stopping fluvoxamine and commencing a tetracyclic antidepressant
- Propranolol – increased propranolol plasma level
- Warfarin – increased warfarin plasma level

Monoamine oxidase inhibitors

Indications

Depressive illness, especially if:

- Anxiety symptoms are present
- Phobic symptoms are present
- Treatment with other types of antidepressant has failed

Also may be of value in the following conditions:

- Agoraphobia
- Chronic facial pain

- Encapsulated delusions of parasitic infestation
- Obsessive compulsive neurosis

Types

- Hydrazine
  - iproniazid
  - isocarboxazid
  - phenelzine
- Non-hydrazine
  - tranylcypromine

Contraindications

- Cardiovascular disease
- Cerebrovascular disease
- Children
- Epilepsy
- Hepatic disease
- Phaeochromocytoma

- In addition, tranylcypromine is also contraindicated in hyper-thyroidism
- Caution is required in the elderly
- Sudden withdrawal should be avoided

Side-effects

Severe hypertensive reactions occur if certain drugs or foods are taken which contain amines, especially tyramine, that may interact with monoamine oxidase inhibitors. Pharmacies and doctors should give patients being treated with monoamine oxidase inhibitors treatment cards listing precautions that need to be taken.

Foods that may interact with MAOIs include:

- Cheese, except
  - cottage cheese
  - cream cheese
- Meat and yeast extracts (e.g. Bovril, Marmite, Oxo)
- Alcohol (particularly Chianti)
- Non-fresh fish, meat, or poultry
- Offal
- Avocado
- Banana skins

- Broad bean pods
- Caviar
- Herring (pickled or smoked)

Neuropsychiatric
- Blurred vision
- Drowsiness
- Insomnia (especially with tranylcypromine, hence the last dose should not be administered later than the early afternoon)
- Tremor

Less commonly
- Ataxia
- Confusional state
- Epilepsy
- Excitement
- Hallucinations
- Hyperreflexia
- Insomnia
- Loss of appetite
- Muscular spasm
- Neck rigidity
- Nightmares
- Oculomotor paralysis
- Paraesthesia
- Peripheral neuropathy
- Worsening or precipitation of
  ○ hypomania and mania
  ○ migraine
  ○ schizophrenia

Cardiac
- Postural hypotension
- Hypertensive crisis can occur if certain drugs or foods are taken which contain amines, especially tyramine, leading to the following:
  ○ hypertension
  ○ headache (often throbbing and occipital, and may radiate frontally)
  ○ throbbing and stiffness in the neck
  ○ palpitations
  ○ multiple extrasystoles with bradycardia or tachycardia
  ○ substernal pain
  ○ nausea and vomiting

o pallor
o sweating
o flushing, photophobia and mydriasis may follow the above
  features
o intracranial haemorrhage which may lead to
  – hemiparesis
  – hemiplegia
  – death

Gastrointestinal
● Constipation
● Dry mouth
● Nausea

Haematological (uncommon)
● Leucopenia

Sexual
● Erectile dysfunction
● Impairment of ejaculation
● Impairment of orgasm

Urinary
● Hesitancy
● Retention

Others (mostly occurring only rarely)
● Blood sugar changes
● Blood dyscrasias
● Dependence on tranylcypromine
● Dermatological disorders
● Hepatocellular jaundice
● Oedema
● Purpura
● Sweating

Interactions with other drugs

Note that foods that may interact with monoamine oxidase
inhibitors are summarized above.

At least 14 days should elapse between stopping a monoamine
oxidase inhibitor and commencing any of the following drugs
which could induce a hypertensive crisis:
● Adrenaline

- Dexamphetamine
- Levodopa
- Metaraminol
- Noradrenaline
- Pemoline

- Dextromethorphan
- Ephedrine
- Phenylephrine
- Phenylethylamine
- Phenylpropranolamine
- Pseudoephedrine

- Fluvoxamine
- Tricyclic antidepressants

- Diethylpropion
- Fenfluramine
- Mazindol
- Phentermine

Phenothiazines: aliphatic side chain

Indications

- Schizophrenia and other psychoses
- Tranquillization and emergency control in disturbed behaviour
- Severe anxiety
- Promotion of weight gain in anorexia nervosa

Types

- Chlorpromazine
- Promazine

Contraindications

- Bone marrow depression
- Angle-closure glaucoma
- CNS depressant induced coma

- Caution is required in the following:
  - pregnancy
  - breast feeding should be suspended
  - hepatic dysfunction
  - renal dysfunction

- ○ epilepsy
- ○ hypothyroidism
- ○ Parkinson's disease
- ○ cardiac failure
- ○ phaeochromocytoma
- ○ myasthenia gravis
- ○ prostatic hypertrophy
- ○ respiratory disease
- ○ acute infections
- ○ a history of jaundice
- ○ leucopenia
- Should also be used with caution in the elderly, particularly in very hot or very cold weather, as there is a risk of hyperthermia or hypothermia, respectively

Side-effects

Cardiovascular
- Hypotension, usually postural
- Cardiac arrhythmias
- ECG changes (including increased QT interval, ST depression, T wave changes)

Respiratory
- Depression

Neurological
- Acute dystonias or dyskinesias
- Akathisia
- Parkinsonism
- Tardive dyskinesia

Anticholinergic symptoms
As with tricyclic antidepressants – see above.

Endocrine
- Hyperprolactinaemia, leading to galactorrhoea, gynaecomastia and menstrual disturbances
- Impotence
- Weight gain

Sensitivity reactions
- Leucopenia
- Leucocytosis

- Agranulocytosis
- Haemolytic anaemia
- Jaundice
- Photosensitization
- Contact sensitization
- Rashes

Others
- Hypothermia/hyperthermia
- Drowsiness
- Apathy
- Insomnia
- Nightmares
- Depression or occasionally agitation
- Neuroleptic malignant syndrome (this can occur with any neuroleptic)
- In those taking chlorpromazine continuously for years, ocular changes (including corneal and lens opacities) and the development of a metallic mauve-grey pigmentation of the skin, conjunctiva, cornea and retina have been noted

Interactions with other drugs

- Tricyclic antidepressants – increased side-effects
- Antiepileptics – antagonism of antiepileptic action
- Drugs for parkinsonism
  - antagonism of antiparkinsonian actions
  - with anticholinergic, antiparkinsonian drugs there is an increase in anticholinergic side-effects
- Antihypertensives – increased hypotensive effect may occur with most antihypertensives (especially α-adrenoceptor antagonists)
- Ethanol, barbiturates and other sedatives
  - increased CNS depressant action of phenothiazines
  - may lead to respiratory depression
- Interference with the absorption of phenothiazines may be caused by
  - antacids
  - antiparkinsonian agents
  - lithium
- Hypoglycaemic agents – the hypoglycaemic response is reduced by high doses of chlorpromazine
- Chlorpromazine may antagonize the action of drugs such as
  - adrenaline
  - amphetamine

○ clonidine
○ guanethidine
○ levodopa
- The simultaneous administration of desferrioxamine and prochlorperazine may lead to a transient metabolic encephalopathy

Phenothiazines: piperidine side chain

This group includes:

- Mesoridazine
- Pericyazine
- Thioridazine

The indications are similar to those for chlorpromazine, with thioridazine often being used in agitation.

Other details are also similar to those for chlorpromazine, with the following important differences:

- Thioridazine is less sedating
- Extrapyramidal symptoms and hypothermia are much less common
- Thioridazine is more likely to cause hypotension
- Thioridazine may cause retrograde ejaculation
- In high doses thioridazine may cause pigmentary retinopathy

Phenothiazines: piperazine side chain

This group includes:

- Fluphenazine
- Perphenazine
- Prochlorperazine
- Trifluoperazine

There are, in general, fewer anticholinergic and sedative effects with this group compared with the two groups above. However, this group tends to have greater extrapyramidal side-effects than the other two groups.

Other antipsychotics

The butyrophenones include:

- Benperidol
- Droperidol

- Haloperidol
- Trifluperidol

Haloperidol has fewer anticholinergic, hypotensive and sedative effects than chlorpromazine, but greater extrapyramidal side-effects (particularly akathisia and dystonic reactions – especially in hyperthyroidism). Haloperidol is more likely to be used in mania, and is also indicated in the Gilles de la Tourette syndrome.

The diphenylbutylpiperidines include:

- Fluspirilene
- Pimozide

They are less sedating than chlorpromazine and have a prolonged action.

The thioxanthenes include:

- Flupenthixol
- Zuclopenthixol

Flupenthixol is less sedating than chlorpromazine, with greater extrapyramidal side-effects. It is also thought to have some antidepressant actions.

Sulpiride is a substituted benzamide which may have fewer extrapyramidal side-effects than chlorpromazine and which may be less likely to cause tardive dyskinesia. In addition to the contraindications to chlorpromazine, sulpiride is also contraindicated in phaeochromocytoma, and a reduced dosage should be used in renal impairment.

Lithium

Indications

- Treatment of mania
- Prophylaxis of recurrent bipolar and unipolar disorder
- Aggressive or self-mutilating behaviour
- Alcoholism

Contraindications

- Renal insufficiency
- Cardiovascular insufficiency
- Addison's disease
- Untreated hypothyroidism

Caution is required in

- Pregnancy
- Breast feeding
- Myasthenia gravis

It is important to monitor plasma lithium levels and thyroid function regularly.

Intake of fluid and sodium must be adequate while on lithium treatment.

A reduced dose is used in the elderly.

Side-effects

- Gastrointestinal effects, including:
  - nausea
  - vomiting
  - diarrhoea
- Fine tremor
- Dry mouth, polyuria and polydipsia
- Vertigo, muscle weakness and a dazed feeling (especially initially)
- Weight gain and oedema (should not be treated with diuretics)

Rarer side-effects include:

- Aggravation of dermatological conditions such as acne, psoriasis, leg ulcers and rashes
- Hypercalcaemia
- Hypermagnesaemia
- Hyperparathyroidism
- Hypokalaemia
- Raised concentration of antidiuretic hormone

Signs of lithium intoxication:
- Gastrointestinal
  - anorexia
  - diarrhoea
  - vomiting
- Central nervous system
  - blurred vision
  - muscle weakness and twitching
  - lack of coordination
  - mild drowsiness and sluggishness progressing to giddiness with ataxia
  - tinnitus

- o dysarthria
- o coarse tremor

At plasma levels above 2 mM: hyperreflexia and hyperextension of limbs, toxic psychoses, convulsions, syncope, oliguria, circulatory failure, coma and death.

Side-effects following long-term treatment
- Thyroid function disturbances
  - o goitre
  - o hypothyroidism
  - o hyperthyroidism
- Memory impairment
- Nephrotoxicity
  - o up to one-third of patients develop polyuria
  - o histological and functional renal changes may occur, and therefore it is recommended that after a period of 3–5 years patients should be continued on maintenance lithium treatment only if, on assessment, benefit persists
- Cardiovascular
  - o T wave flattening on ECG
  - o arrhythmias

Interactions with other drugs
- Diuretics and in sodium depletion
  - o reduced lithium clearance leading to potentiation of lithium
  - o loop diuretics such as frusemide are safer than thiazide diuretics
- Acetazolamide, sodium bicarbonate, theophylline – increased lithium excretion
- Amiloride
  - o antagonism of lithium-induced polyuria
  - o lithium clearance is not reduced
- Antidiabetic agents – lithium may impair glucose tolerance
- Carbamazepine, diltiazem, methyldopa, phenytoin, verapamil – can cause CNS toxicity without increasing plasma concentration
- Diazepam – hypothermia has been reported (very rarely)
- Diclofenac, ibuprofen, indomethacin, mefanamic acid, naproxen, phenylbutazone, piroxicam – potentiation of lithium
- Enalapril – increased plasma lithium concentration
- Haloperidol, metoclopramide, phenothiazine derivatives – increased risk of extrapyramidal side-effects

- Muscle relaxants – potentiation of the muscle relaxants
- Neostigmine, pyridostigmine – lithium may antagonize the actions of neostigmine and pyridostigmine and cause deterioration in myasthenia gravis
- Steroids – steroids may alter lithium excretion by altering electrolyte balance

Carbamazepine

Indications

- All types of epilepsy apart from absence seizures
- Prophylaxis of manic depressive psychosis in lithium resistant patients
- The paroxysmal pain of trigeminal neuralgia

Contraindications

- Previous drug sensitivity to carbamazepine
- Atrioventricular conduction abnormalities (unless paced)
- Porphyrias
- Should not be administered with or within 2 weeks of cessation of MAOI therapy

Caution is required in:

- Hepatic impairment
- Pregnancy
- Breast feeding

Monitoring of plasma levels may be of help in determining optimum dosage.

It is recommended that during therapy plasma folic acid levels are regularly measured. This also applies to the other anticonvulsants that are discussed below.

Side-effects

- Dizziness
- Diplopia (usually dose dependent)
- Drowsiness
- Dry mouth, diarrhoea, nausea, vomiting
- Hyponatraemia (on high dosage), oedema
- Generalized erythematous rash (in 3% of patients)
- Blood disorders, including leucopenia (rare)

Interactions with other drugs

- Drugs whose activity may be reduced by carbamazepine including:
  - warfarin and nicoumalone
  - theophylline
  - haloperidol
  - clonazepam
  - ethosuximide
  - doxycycline
  - thyroxine
  - corticosteroids
  - oral contraceptives
- Drugs which may elevate carbamazepine levels including:
  - macrolide antibiotics (e.g. erythromycin)
  - isoniazid
  - some calcium antagonists (such as verapamil and diltiazem)
  - dextropropoxyphene
  - viloxazine
  - cimetidine
  - danazol
- Lithium – see above
  MAOIs – see above

Ethosuximide

Indications

- Absence seizures

Contraindications

- Porphyrias

Caution – see under carbamazepine

Side-effects

- Gastrointestinal effects
- Drowsiness, ataxia, dizziness
- Headache
- Depression
- Mild euphoria

Rare side-effects include psychotic states, blood disorders and rashes.

Interactions with other drugs

- Carbamazepine – see above
- Drugs may elevate ethosuximide levels including:
  - isoniazid
  - sodium valproate

Phenobarbitone

Indications

- All types of epilepsy apart from absence seizures
- Occasionally used in status epilepticus but is not the drug of choice

Contraindications

- Porphyrias

Caution is required in:

- Hepatic or renal impairment
- Pregnancy
- Breast feeding
- The elderly and children
- Respiratory depression

Sudden withdrawal should be avoided.

Side-effects

- Drowsiness, lethargy
- Ataxia
- Depression
- Dermatological reactions
- Megaloblastic anaemia

In the elderly there may be paradoxical excitement and confusion. Hyperkinesia may occur in children.

Interactions with other drugs

- Drugs whose activity may be reduced by phenobarbitone including:
  - warfarin and nicoumalone
  - digitoxin

- ○ disopyramide, quinidine
- ○ theophylline
- ○ tricyclic antidepressants
- ○ clonazepam
- ○ chloramphenicol, doxycycline, metronidazole, griseofulvin
- ○ corticosteroids
- ○ oral contraceptives
- ○ cyclosporin
- Drugs which may cause increased sedation including:
  - ○ phenytoin
  - ○ sodium valproate

Phenytoin

Indications

- All types of epilepsy apart from absence seizures

Contraindications

- Porphyrias

Caution is required in:
- Hepatic impairment
- Pregnancy

Should be introduced gradually with small increments being made until therapeutic plasma levels (if facilities are available), control or toxic effects appear.

Sudden withdrawals should be avoided.

Side-effects

During initial treatment, the following side-effects, which often subside with continued use, may occur:

- Nausea, vomiting
- Transient nervousness
- Insomnia
- Weight loss
- Dizziness, headache

Signs of overdosage:
- Ataxia
- Slurred speech
- Blurred vision
- Nystagmus

Other side-effects:
- Coarse facies, dermatological eruptions, acne, hirsutism
- Pyrexia
- Hepatitis
- Lupus erythematosus, erythema multiforme
- Lymphadenopathy
- Gingival hypertrophy and tenderness
- Haematological effects, including
  - agranulocytosis
  - aplastic anaemia
  - leucopenia
  - megaloblastic anaemia
  - thrombocytopenia
- Hypocalcaemia

Interactions with other drugs

- Drugs whose activity may be reduced by phenytoin including:
  - warfarin and nicoumalone (potentiation is also reported)
  - digitoxin
  - disopyramide, quinidine
  - theophylline
  - tricyclic antidepressants
  - clonazepam
  - doxycycline, ketoconazole
  - thyroxine
  - corticosteroids
  - oral contraceptives
  - cyclosporin
- Drugs which may potentiate phenytoin including:
  - amiodarone
  - aspirin, azapropazone, phenylbutazone
  - chloramphenicol, co-trimoxazole, isoniazid, ketoconazole, metronidazole, miconazole
  - cimetidine
  - diazepam
  - disulfiram
  - influenza vaccine
  - sodium valproate
  - sulphinpyrazone
  - viloxazine
- Drugs which may reduce the plasma level of phenytoin including:
  - folic acid
  - rifampicin

- Sucralfate – causes reduced absorption of phenytoin
- Lithium and phenobarbitone – see above

Sodium valproate

Indications

- All forms of epilepsy

Contraindications

- Acute hepatic disease

Caution is required in:

- Hepatic impairment
- Pregnancy
- Breast feeding
- Children

Hepatic function should be monitored in patients most at risk. Platelet function should be monitored prior to major surgery. Note that sodium valproate may give a false positive result in a urine ketone test.

Side-effects

- Nausea
- Increased appetite, weight gain
- Hyperammonaemia
- Hair loss (transient)
- Oedema
- Impaired hepatic function (may rarely progress to fatal hepatic failure)
- Inhibition of platelet aggregation, thrombocytopenia
- Pancreatitis (rare – in acute abdominal pain the plasma amylase should therefore be measured)

Treatment should be stopped immediately should any of the following occur:

- Vomiting
- Drowsiness
- Anorexia
- Jaundice
- Loss of seizure control

Interactions with other drugs

- Drugs may reduce the plasma level of sodium valproate including:
  - carbamazepine
  - phenobarbitone
  - phenytoin
  - primidone
- Sodium valproate may also interact with phenobarbitone and primidone to cause increased sedation
- Ethosuximide – see above

Specimen MCQ

The following is Question 21 taken from page 11 of the *Report to the Court of Electors, The Royal College of Psychiatrists Working Party for Review of the MRCPsych*. Responsibility for the answers is taken by the authors.

A patient being treated with a monoamine oxidase inhibitor should not eat:

A. Broad beans removed from their pods
B. Cottage cheese
C. Pickled herrings
D. Fresh calf liver
E. Well-hung pheasant

Answers

A. FALSE It is the broad bean pods which should not be eaten
B. FALSE Cottage and cream cheese may be eaten
C. TRUE
D. FALSE
E. TRUE

Bibliography

Berrios, G.E. and Dowson, J.H. (editors) (1983) *Treatment and Management in Adult Psychiatry*. London: Baillière Tindall.
British Medical Association and The Pharmaceutical Press (1989) *British National Formulary*, No. 17. British Medical Association and The Pharmaceutical Press, London.
Crammer, J.L., Barraclough, B. and Heine, B. (1978) *The Use of Drugs in Psychiatry*. London: Gaskell.

Crawford, R. and Silverstone, T. (1987) *Carbamazepine in Affective Disorder.* London: Clinical Neuroscience Publishers.

Gelder, M., Gath, D. and Mayou, R. (1989) *Oxford Textbook of Psychiatry,* 2nd edition. Oxford: Oxford University Press.

Kaplan, H.I. and Sadock, B.J. (editors) (1989) *Comprehensive Textbook of Psychiatry,* 5th edition. Baltimore: Williams and Wilkins.

Kendell, R.E. and Zealley, A.K. (editors) (1988) *Companion to Psychiatric Studies,* 4th edition. Edinburgh: Churchill Livingstone.

McGuffin, P., Shanks, M.F. and Hodgson, R.J. (1984) *The Scientific Principles of Psychopathology.* London: Grune and Stratton.

Rogers, H.J. and Spector, R.G. (1984) *Aids to Clinical Pharmacology and Therapeutics.* Edinburgh: Churchill Livingstone.

Silverstone, T. and Turner, P. (1978) *Drug Treatment in Psychiatry.* London: Routledge and Kegan Paul.

The Association of the British Pharmaceutical Industry (1988) *ABPI Data Sheet Compendium 1989–90.* London: Datapharm Publications.

The Royal College of Psychiatrists (1985) *Report to the Court of Electors, The Royal College of Psychiatrists Working Party for Review of the MRCPsych.* London: The Royal College of Psychiatrists.

The Royal College of Psychiatrists (1987) *General Information and Regulations for the MRCPsych Examinations,* 8th revision. London: The Royal College of Psychiatrists.

Tyrer, P. (editor) (1982) *Drugs in Psychiatric Practice.* London: Butterworths.

Chapter 6

Methods of clinical assessment in psychiatry

Syllabus requirements

The candidate will be expected to have the requisite knowledge about practical procedures. Thus he or she will be required to understand the principles underlying the clinical methods of psychiatry: the establishing of a satisfactory working relationship with the patient, the eliciting of accurate information under the several headings of the psychiatric history, the procedures for examining the patient's mental state and related abnormalities on physical examination, and the integrating of this information in clinical assessment with recognition of the need for further examination, information and/or investigations.

Textbooks are clearly not an adequate substitute for experience in clerking psychiatric patients. Candidates would therefore do well to practise and refine their clinical skills prior to the examination. Note that in the MRCPsych Part I Examination, the clinical examination must be passed in order to pass the whole examination. A good pass in this part of the examination may be sufficient to allow a candidate who has narrowly failed in the multiple choice paper to pass overall. However, the converse is not true, i.e. however well a candidate does on the multiple choice paper, failing the clinical examination will result in failure of the whole MRCPsych Part I Examination.

The clinical examination

The MRCPsych Part I Clinical Examination will test basic clinical skills of psychiatric assessment: the ability to relate to the patient, to take a history and examine the mental state, and to exercise judgement in bringing the relevant information together to make a succinct and accurate assessment. A detailed plan of management is not required. (The latter is tested in the Part II Examination.)

Candidates will be expected to examine a case or cases which may be drawn from any aspect of adult general psychiatry for 50 minutes. During the 30 minute interview with a pair of Examiners, candidates are expected to further interview the patient for about 10 minutes in the presence of the Examiners. The main areas of assessment are the candidate's ability to establish a satisfactory relationship with the patient, take a full psychiatric history, carry out an accurate mental state examination, make appropriate deductions from the information available to him or her, and come to a conclusion concerning the diagnosis and differential diagnosis of the disorder(s) from which the patient is suffering.

Candidates will not be expected to carry out a physical examination as a routine, but a selective examination should be undertaken if this seems to be called for by observations made during the interview. These may include examination of the pulse, blood pressure, fundi, extrapyramidal system, etc. The necessary instruments and facilities will be available during the Clinical Examination.

History

- Name, age, date of admission (if applicable), etc.
- Reason(s) for referral and source of referral
- History of presenting illness
  - details of each symptom
  - effects of the symptoms on social functioning, etc.
  - treatment received
- If appropriate, the effects of the illness on the following can be noted: sleep (e.g. early morning wakening, initial insomnia, broken sleep); appetite; weight; energy; hobbies; concentration; thoughts about the future, guilt feelings; libido; menstrual function (if appropriate)
- Diurnal variation of mood, tearfulness, suicidal feelings, etc., during the illness, can also be enquired about.
- Family history
  - Parental and sibling details including
    - current age or age at death
    - occupation
    - health
    - relationship with patient
  - social aspects
- Family psychiatric history
- Personal history
  - date of birth

- o place of birth
- o abnormalities prior to or at birth
- o early development (milestones)
- o childhood health (including any history of 'nervous problems')
- o schooling (including relationship with others and qualifications)
- o higher education
- o occupations
- o menstrual history (if appropriate)
- o psychosexual and marital history
- o occupation of spouse and current social situation
- o details of children (if appropriate)
- Past medical history
- Past psychiatric history
  - o nature of illness(es)
  - o duration of illness(es)
  - o hospital(s) attended
  - o treatment(s) received
- Forensic history
- Drug history – include history of alcohol intake, tobacco use, and any history of illicit drug abuse
- Premorbid personality
  - o predominant mood
  - o relationships
  - o character
  - o attitudes, religion

Qualities of a good history

In the Psychiatric Examination situation, some of the qualities that are looked for in the history include the following:

- The history should be systematic with the appropriate use of headings such as those given above
- The history should be comprehensive without being overinclusive. It should give only the positive features, together with any relevant negative findings
- The history should be coherent and internally consistent
- The history should demonstrate that the candidate has an appropriate sense of priorities and clinical relevance. Unnecessary details should be avoided
- The history should be multidimensional in its approach, taking note of relevant psychological and social aspects

- The history should distinguish clearly between fact and opinion
- The history should be accurate. This helps to demonstrate good communication between the candidate and the patient
- The history should pay due attention to the problem of reliability. It may be useful to mention the need to seek further clarification of aspects of the history from other informants

Mental state examination

Appearance

- General appearance
- Body build (e.g. recent weight loss?)
- Clothing
- Facial appearance
- Posture

Behaviour

- Movements (including gait)
- Eye contact
- Social behaviour
- Motor disorders, e.g.
  - ambitendence
  - echopraxia
  - negativism
  - posturing
  - stereotypies
  - tardive dyskinesia
  - waxy flexibility (also called flexibilitas cerea)

Speech

- Rate
- Quantity
- Accent
- Flow
- The presence of neologisms

Disorders of flow include:

- Flight of ideas
- Sudden interruptions
- Those seen in thought disorder

It may be useful to record a sample of the patient's speech.

Mood

There is some overlap here with the history of the presenting illness, although in the mental state examination the candidate will be examining the mood of the patient at the time of the assessment itself:

- Appropriateness
- Sleep
- Appetite
- Energy
- Libido
- Feelings of guilt
- Hopelessness
- Suicidal thoughts
- Anxiety symptoms and thoughts
- Elation
- Blunting of affect
- etc.

It is not necessary to mention all the physiological disturbances that can accompany depressed mood if they are not relevant to the case. What is needed is an assessment of the objective and subjective aspects of the mood. Some psychiatrists also include rapport under mood.

Rapport

Depersonalization and derealization

Obsessional phenomena

Abnormal beliefs

- Ideas of reference
- Overvalued ideas
- Primary delusions
- Secondary delusions
- Delusional perception
- Delusional mood

Delusions include the following types:

- Persecutory
- Grandiose
- Hypochondriacal
- Nihilistic
- Amorous

- Religious
- Thought insertion
- Thought broadcasting
- Thought withdrawal
- Delusions of control
- Delusions of reference
- Delusions of guilt
- Delusions of jealousy

Illusions and hallucinations

- Hallucinations may be true or dissociative
- Modalities include:
  - auditory
  - visual
  - tactile
  - gustatory
  - olfactory
- Hypnagogic hallucinations
- Hypnopompic hallucinations

Thought content (not included above)

- Preoccupations
- Phobias
- (Suicidal thoughts, if not already mentioned under the heading of mood)
- Homicidal thoughts
- Recurrent ideas about hypochondriacal symptomatology
- Abstract thinking

Orientation

- Time
- Place
- Person

Memory

- Registration and immediate recall
- Short-term memory
- Memory for recent events
- Long-term memory

Attention and concentration

General information and intelligence

Insight

Does the patient:
- Recognize that he or she is ill?
- Accept that he or she has a psychiatric illness?
- Accept that psychiatric treatment is necessary?

Clinical skills

The 30 minutes spent with the examiners in the MRCPsych Part I Clinical Examination are split into three periods of approximately 10 minutes, as follows:

- First 10-minute period: candidate presents his or her assessment
- Second 10-minute period: candidate interviews the patient in the presence of the examiners
- Third 10-minute period: candidate discusses his or her findings with the examiners

In assessing a candidate's clinical skills, examiners may play particular attention to the candidate's technique, and also his or her qualities.

Criteria used to assess whether a candidate exhibits a good clinical technique can include whether he or she:

- is systematic
- is comprehensive
- is flexible
- is goal directed
- demonstrates sensitive control of the interview
- allows the patient to talk
- uses appropriate forms of questions (open rather than leading)
- uses summary statements and clarification

Important qualities for a candidate to develop and to demonstrate in a clinical examination include being:

- considerate
- tactful
- sensitive to the patient's problem(s) and mental state
- empathic
- objective
- confident

Objectivity includes the ability to explore all the relevant theories without the premature closure of options.

In addition, a candidate should demonstrate self-control. This may be evidenced by his or her ability to tolerate fustration, provocation, ambiguity and uncertainty.

Another mark of a good candidate is his or her ability to discuss any relevant psychodynamic factors in an appropriate way. A consideration of such factors is often of a poor standard in clinical psychiatric examinations, and the reader is referred to Chapter 8 for further details.

Physical examination

There is usually insufficient time for a full physical examination in this part of the Examination. However, it is usually possible to check the patient's pulse, blood pressure, fundi, etc. Useful details are to be found in textbooks of neurology and medicine.

Organic syndrome

If an organic syndrome is suspected a full neurological examination should be performed (time permitting).

Apraxia

- Constructional apraxia – the patient is asked to construct a star or other figure out of matchsticks, or else to draw it
- Dressing apraxia – the patient can be asked to put on items of his or her clothing
- Ideomotor apraxia – the patient is asked to carry out increasingly difficult tasks, for example involving touching parts of his or her face with specified fingers

Agnosia

- Agraphognosia/agraphaesthesia – the patient is asked to identify numbers or letters traced on to his or her palms
- Anosognosia – e.g. the patient is unaware of left-sided weakness and sensory inattention following a right parietal lesion
- Astereognosia – the patient, with eyes closed, is asked to identify objects such as coins placed in his or her hand
- Finger agnosia – the patient, with eyes closed, is asked to identify which of his or her fingers has been touched
- Topognosia – the patient is asked to locate the position of an object on his or her skin

Language ability

- Dysarthria – the patient is asked to repeat a phrase such as 'West Register Street' or 'The Leith police dismisseth us'
- Expressive or motor aphasia
  - the patient is asked to talk about his or her hobbies
  - the patient is asked to name objects
  - the patient is asked to write to dictation
  - the patient is asked to write a passage spontaneously
- Receptive or sensory aphasia
  - the patient is asked to read a passage
  - the patient is asked to explain the passage
  - the patient is asked to respond to commands
- Global aphasia – a combination of expressive and receptive aphasic difficulties

Bibliography

Bannister, R. (1985) *Brain's Clinical Neurology*, 6th edition. Oxford: Oxford University Press.

Gelder, M., Gath, D. and Mayou, R. (1989) *Oxford Textbook of Psychiatry*, 2nd edition. Oxford: Oxford University Press.

Holden, N. (1987) *Examination Technique in Psychiatry*. London: Edward Arnold.

Institute of Psychiatry (1973) *Notes on Eliciting and Recording Clinical Information*. Oxford: Oxford University Press.

Kaplan, H.I. and Sadock, B.J. (editors) (1989) *Comprehensive Textbook of Psychiatry*, 5th edition. Baltimore: Williams and Wilkins.

Kendell, R.E. and Zealley, A.K. (editors) (1988) *Companion to Psychiatric Studies*, 4th edition. Edinburgh: Churchill Livingstone.

Leff, J.P. and Isaacs, A.D. (1981) *Psychiatric Examination in Clinical Practice*. Oxford: Blackwell Scientific.

Lishman, W.A. (1987) *Organic Psychiatry: The Psychological Consequences of Cerebral Disorder*, 2nd edition. Oxford: Blackwell Scientific.

McGuffin, P. and Greer, S. (1987) *A Psychiatric Catechism*. London: Edward Arnold.

Sims, A.C.P. (1985) *Symptoms in the Mind*. London: Baillière Tindall.

The Royal College of Psychiatrists (1985) *Report to the Court of Electors, The Royal College of Psychiatrists Working Party for Review of the MRCPsych*. London: The Royal College of Psychiatrists.

The Royal College of Psychiatrists (1987) *General Information and Regulations for the MRCPsych Examinations*, 8th revision. London: The Royal College of Psychiatrists.

Walton, J. (1985) *Brain's Diseases of the Nervous System*, 9th edition. Oxford: Oxford University Press.

Wilkinson, I.M.S. (1988) *Essential Neurology*. Oxford: Blackwell Scientific Publications.

Chapter 7

Descriptive psychopathology

Syllabus requirements

The candidate will be expected to have a basic knowledge of the phenomenology of psychiatry and the ways in which symptoms and signs are expressed and experienced.

Once again the need for regular practice of clinical skills cannot be overemphasized, and this is the best method by which to understand and learn 'the ways in which symptoms and signs are expressed and experienced'. This chapter concentrates on the required basic knowledge of the phenomenology of psychiatry although here again frequent practice of clinical skills will be found to be of great value.

Disorders of general behaviour

Underactivity

Depressive retardation
- Prominent psychomotor retardation
- Extreme form merges with depressive stupor

Stupor
The patient shows lack of reaction to and unawareness of the environment, and can be aroused only by considerable stimulation.

Main types:

- Catatonic
- Depressive
- Organic
- hysterical
Stupor can also be classified under disorders of consciousness (see below).

Obsessional slowness
- Primary

- Secondary to
  - repeated doubts
  - compulsive rituals

Overactivity

Psychomotor agitation
- Excess overactivity and restlessness
- Usually unproductive
- Response to emotional tension

Hyperkinesis
- May be seen in children

Somnambulism
- Complex sequence of behaviours is carried out by a person who rises from sleep and is not fully aware of his or her surroundings at the time

Compulsion
- Repetitive and stereotyped seemingly purposeful behaviour
- Also known as compulsive rituals
- May alternatively be classified with obsessions (see below) although strictly speaking compulsions are the motor component of obsessional thoughts

- Types include:
  - checking rituals
  - cleaning rituals
  - counting rituals
  - dressing rituals
  - dipsomania (compulsion to drink)
  - kleptomania (compulsion to steal)
  - nymphomania (compulsive need to engage in coitus in the female)
  - satyriasis (compulsive need to engage in coitus in the male)
  - trichotillomania (compulsion to pull one's hair out)

Abnormal movements

Ambitendence
- Alternation between opposite movements

Echopraxia
- Pathological automatic imitation of another person's movements
- Occurs even when patient asked not to

Mannerisms
- Repeated involuntary movements that appear to be goal directed

Negativism
- Motiveless resistance to instructions and to attempts to be moved

Posturing
- Adoption of inappropriate or bizarre bodily posture continuously for a substantial period of time

Stereotypies
- Repeated regular fixed pattern of movement (or speech) which is not goal directed

Tics
- Repeated irregular movements
- Involves a muscle group

Waxy flexibility
- Patient's limbs can be 'moulded' into a position and remain fixed for long periods of time
- Also known as cerea flexibilitas

Disorders of speech

Aphasia

Receptive aphasia
- Difficulty in comprehending word meanings
- Also known as sensory aphasia and Wernicke's fluent aphasia
- Types include
  - agnosic alexia (words can be seen but not read)
  - pure word deafness (words that are heard cannot be comprehended)
  - visual asymbolia (patient can transcribe but has difficulty in reading)

Intermediate aphasia
Types include:

- Nominal aphasia (difficulty in naming objects)
- Central aphasia (difficulty in arranging words in proper sequence; also known as syntactical aphasia)

Expressive aphasia
- Difficulty in expressing thoughts in words but understanding remains
- Also known as motor aphasia and Broca's nonfluent aphasia

Global aphasia
- Grossly non-fluent aphasia and severe fluent aphasia both present at the same time

Jargon aphasia
- Incoherent meaningless neologistic speech

Other speech disorders

Stammering and stuttering

Mutism
- Complete loss of speech

Vorbeireden
- Also known as talking past the point
- Answers to questions, although clearly incorrect, demonstrate that the question was understood

Neologisms
- New words constructed by the patient or everyday words used in a special way by the patient

Schizophasia
- Incoherent and incomprehensible mixture of words and phrases
- Also known as word salad and speech confusion

Pressure of speech
- Increased amount and rate of speech
- Difficult to interrupt

Dysprosody
- Loss of the normal melody of speech

Logorrhoea
- Speech fluent and rambling with many words
- Also known as volubility

Dysarthria
- Difficulty in articulation of speech

Poverty of speech
- Restricted amount of speech
- Patient may reply to questions with monosyllabic answers

Disorders of emotion

Affect

According to DSM-III-R, the affect refers to 'a pattern of observable behaviours that is the expression of a subjectively experienced feeling state (emotion)...Affect is variable over time, in response to changing emotional states, whereas mood refers to a pervasive and sustained emotion.'

Inappropriate
- The affect is inappropriate to the thought or speech it accompanies

Blunted
- Externalized feeling tone is severely reduced

Flat
- Total or almost total absence of signs of expression of affect

Labile
- Labile emotional feeling tone
- Not related to environmental stimuli

Mood

DSM-III-R defines mood as 'a pervasive and sustained emotion that, in the extreme, markedly colours the person's perception of the world'.

Alexithymia
- Difficulty in being aware of or describing the emotions one feels

Anhedonia
- Loss of ability to enjoy regular and pleasurable activities with loss of interest in them

Depression

Dysphoric mood
- An unpleasant mood

Ecstasy
- A feeling of intense rapture

Elevated mood
- A mood more cheerful than normal
- Not necessarily pathological

Euphoric mood
- Exaggerated feeling of well-being
- Pathological

Expansive mood
- Feelings are expressed without restraint
- Patient may overestimate his or her importance or significance

Grief
- In normal grief or mourning the sadness is appropriate to the loss

Irritable mood
- Patient is easily annoyed and provoked to anger

Mood swings

Other emotions

Agitation
- Excessive motor activity associated with a feeling of inner tension

Ambivalence
- Simultaneous presence of opposing impulses towards the same thing

Anxiety
- Feeling of apprehension, tension, or uneasiness owing to the anticipation of an external or internal danger

Types include:

- Phobia (the focus of the anxiety is avoided; see below under disorders of thought content)
- Free-floating anxiety (anxiety is pervasive and unfocused)
- Panic attacks (anxiety is experienced in acute, episodic, intense attacks and may be accompanied by physiological symptoms)

Apathy
- Loss of emotional tone and ability to feel pleasure, associated with detachment or indifference

Fear
- Anxiety owing to realistic danger that is recognized consciously

Tension
- Unpleasant increase in psychomotor activity

Disorders of thought

Disorders of tempo

Flight of ideas
- Stream of accelerated thoughts with abrupt changes from topic to topic and no central direction
- The connections between thoughts may be based on:
  - chance relationships
  - verbal associations (for example, alliteration and assonance)
  - clang associations
  - distracting stimuli
  - etc.

Inhibition or retardation of thinking
- Train of thought is slowed down
- Lack of elaboration of ideas
- May be part of a generalized psychomotor retardation

Circumstantiality
- Thinking appears slow with the incorporation of unnecessary trivial details
- The goal of thought is finally reached

Disorders of continuity

Perseveration
- Mental operations are continued beyond the point at which they are relevant, thereby preventing progress of thinking

Thought blocking
- Sudden interruption of the train of thought, before it is completed, leaving a 'blank'
- Following a period of silence, the patient cannot recall what he or she had been saying or what he or she had been thinking of saying

Disorders of possession

Obsessions
- According to Schneider 'an obsession occurs, when someone cannot get rid of a content of consciousness, although when it occurs he realizes that it is senseless or at least that it is dominating and persisting without cause'
- Initially resisted
- Themes include
  o fear of causing harm
  o dirt and contamination
  o aggression
  o sexual
  o religious (e.g. blasphemous)
  o etc.
- Compulsions are the motor component of obsessional thoughts and are discussed above

Thought alienation
- According to Fish 'in thought alienation the patient has the experience that his thoughts are under the control of an outside agency or that others are participating in his thinking'

- Types include:
  o thought insertion (patient believes that thoughts are being put into his or her mind by an external agency)
  o thought withdrawal (patient believes that thoughts are being removed from his or her mind by an external agency)
  o thought broadcasting (patient believes that his or her thoughts are being 'read' by others, as if they were being broadcast)

'Made actions'
- Patient feels that his or her free will has been removed and that his or her behaviour is being controlled by an external agency

Disorder of content

Overvalued idea
- An unreasonable and sustained intense preoccupation maintained with less than delusional intensity
- The idea or belief held is demonstrably false and is not one that is normally held by others of the patient's subculture
- There is a marked associated emotional investment

Delusion
According to DSM-III-R a delusion is 'a false personal belief based on incorrect inference about external reality and firmly sustained in spite of what almost everyone else believes and in spite of what constitutes incontrovertible and obvious proof or evidence to the contrary. The belief is not one ordinarily accepted by other members of the person's culture or subculture (i.e. it is not an article of religious faith).'
Types include:

- Bizarre (totally implausible and absurd belief)
- Delusion of doubles (delusional belief that a person known to the patient has been replaced by a double; also known as Capgras' syndrome)
- Delusion of grandeur (exaggerated belief of one's own power and importance)
- Delusion of infidelity (delusional belief that one's spouse or lover is being unfaithful; also known as delusional jealousy and the Othello syndrome)
- Delusion of persecution (delusional belief that one is being persecuted)
- Delusion of poverty (delusional belief that one is in poverty)
- Delusion of reference (delusional belief that the behaviour of others, objects and events such as television and radio broadcasts refer to oneself; when similar thoughts are held but without delusional intensity, they are referred to as ideas of reference)
- Delusion of self-accusation (delusional feeling of guilt)
- Erotomania (delusional belief that another person is deeply in love with the patient; usually occurs in women, with the object often being a man of much higher social status; also known as de Clérambault's syndrome)

- Mood congruent (content of delusion is appropriate to the mood of the patient)
- Mood incongruent (content of delusion is not appropriate to the mood of the patient)
- Nihilistic (delusional belief that others, oneself, or the world does not exist or is about to cease to exist)
- Somatic (delusional belief pertaining to the functioning of one's body)
- Systematized (a group of delusions united by a single theme, or a delusion with multiple elaborations)
- Paranoid (includes delusion of grandeur, delusion of reference, persecutory delusion, and thought alienation; it is derived from the Greek παρα (beside) and νουσ (mind))

Primary delusion
- A delusion arising fully formed without any discernible connection with previous events
- Primary delusions are also known as autochthonous delusions

Delusional mood
- A primary delusion may be preceded by a 'delusion mood' in which the patient is aware of something strange and threatening happening

Delusional perception
- A delusional perception involves a real perception followed by a delusional misinterpretation of that perception

Phobia
- A persistent irrational fear of an activity, object or situation leading to avoidance
- The fear is out of proportion to the real danger and cannot be reasoned away
- The fear is beyond voluntary control

- Types of phobias of external stimuli include:
  - acrophobia (fear of heights)
  - agoraphobia (literally fear of market place; it is a syndrome entailing a generalized high anxiety level and multiple phobic symptoms; it may include fears of crowds, open and closed spaces, shopping, social situations and travelling by bus or train)
  - algophobia (fear of pain)
  - claustrophobia (fear of closed places)

- o simple phobia (fear of discrete objects or situations, e.g. fear of snakes or spiders)
- o social phobia (fear of personal interactions in a public setting, such as a fear of public speaking, eating in public or meeting people)
- o xenophobia (fear of strangers)
- o zoophobia (fear of animals)

- Types of phobias of internal stimuli include:
  - o illness phobias (these overlap with hypochondriasis)
  - o obsessive phobias

Egomania
- Pathological preoccupation with oneself

Hypochondriasis
- Preoccupation with a fear of having a serious illness based not on real organic pathology but rather on an unrealistic interpretation of physical signs or sensations as abnormal

Monomania
- Pathological preoccupation with a single object

Disorders of form

Fusion
- Separate ideas are merged and interweaved

Transitory thinking
- There is disturbance of grammar and syntax

- Types include:
  - o derailment (insertion of inappropriate ideas into the stream of thought leading to a disruption of its continuity)
  - o omission (sudden interruption in the stream of thought)
  - o substitution (minor thought is substituted for a major one)

Desultory thinking
- Inappropriate ideas are inserted into the stream of thought, but the speech is correct in terms of grammar and syntax

Drivelling
- The constituents of an idea are muddled together

Condensation
- Separate ideas are fused to produce an incomprehensible concept (Bleuler)

Overinclusive thinking
- Concept boundaries are broken down giving the concept nebulous boundaries and enlarging it (Cameron)

Disorders of perception

Sensory distortions

Changes in intensity
Types include:
- Hypoaesthesia (reduced intensity of sensations, e.g. hypoacusis)
- Hyperaesthesia (increased intensity of sensations, e.g. hyperacusis)

Changes in quality
- Usually visual distortions
- When perceptions are coloured (e.g. because of toxins) they are named after the colours, for example
  - chloropsia (green)
  - erythropsia (red)
  - xanthopsia (yellow)

Changes in spatial form
Types include:
- Macropsia (objects are seen larger or nearer than is actually the case)
- Micropsia (objects are seen smaller or farther away than is actually the case)

  Also known as dysmegalopsia

Sensory deceptions

Illusion
- False perception of a real external stimulus

Hallucination
- False sensory perception in the absence of a real external stimulus

- Perceived as being located in objective space
- Perceived as having the same realistic qualities as normal perceptions
- Not subject to conscious manipulation
- Only indicate a psychotic disturbance when there is also impaired reality testing

- Types include:
  - auditory
  - autoscopy (the patient sees himself or herself and knows that it is he or she; involves visual, kinaesthetic and somatic sensations; also known as phantom mirror image)
  - extracampine (hallucination occurs outside the patient's sensory field)
  - functional (the stimulus that causes the hallucination is experienced as well as the hallucination)
  - gustatory
  - hallucinosis (hallucinations, which are usually auditory, occur in clear consciousness, and are usually associated with chronic alcohol abuse)
  - hypnagogic (occurs while falling asleep)
  - hypnopompic (occurs while waking from sleep)
  - mood congruent
  - mood incongruent
  - olfactory
  - reflex (a type of synaesthesia; a stimulus in one sensory field leads to a hallucination in another sensory field)
  - somatic (involves the false sensation that things are occurring to or in the patient's body; also known as cenaesthetic hallucination)
  - tactile (also known as haptic hallucination; includes the sensation of insects crawling under the skin, known as formication, and also phantom limb sensations)
  - trailing phenomenon (moving objects are perceived as a series of discrete discontinuous objects; usually associated with hallucinogens)
  - visual

Pseudohallucination
- A form of imagery arising in the mind's subjective inner space
- Lacks the substantiality of normal perceptions
- Occupies subjective space rather than objective space
- Not subject to conscious manipulation

Eidetic image
- Vivid and detailed reproduction of a previous perception, as in a 'photographic memory'
- May be classified as a pseudohallucination

Pareidolia
- Vivid imagery occurs without conscious effort while the person looks at a poorly structured background such as a fire or plain wallpaper

Disorders of intellectual function

Disorders of consciousness

Clouding of consciousness
- Patient is drowsy and does not react completely to stimuli
- There is disturbance of attention, concentration, memory, orientation and thinking

Coma
- Profound unconsciousness with no external evidence of mental activity
- There is little motor activity apart from respiratory movements

Confusion
- Patient is unable to think clearly

Delirium
- A confusional state in which the patient is bewildered, disoriented and restless
- May be associated with fear and hallucinations
- Variations of this syndrome include:
  - oneiroid state (a dream-like state in a patient who is not asleep)
  - torpor (patient is drowsy and easily falls asleep)
  - twilight state (a prolonged oneiroid state of disturbed consciousness with hallucinations).

Disorientation
- Disturbance of orientation in time, place or person.

Fugue
- State of wandering from usual surroundings in which there is also loss of memory

Somnolence
- Abnormal drowsiness

Stupor
Patient appears to be fully conscious often with open eyes that follow objects. However, he or she is mute and immobile, and shows lack of reaction to his or her surroundings.

Disorders of attention

Distractibility
- Attention drawn too frequently to unimportant or irrelevant external stimuli

Selective inattention
- Anxiety provoking stimuli are blocked out

Disorders of memory

Amnesia
- Inability to recall past experiences

- Types include:
  - anterograde
  - retrograde

Hypermnesia
- Degree of retention and recall is exaggerated

Paramnesia
- Distorted recall leading to falsification of memory

- Types include:
  - confabulation (gaps in memory are unconsciously filled with false memories, as in Korsakov's syndrome)
  - déjà entendu (illusion of auditory recognition)
  - déjà pensé (illusion of recognition of a new thought)
  - déjà vu (illusion of visual recognition)
  - fausse reconnaissance (false recognition)
  - jamais vu (illusion of failure to recognize a familiar situation)
  - retrospective falsification (false details are added to the recollection of an otherwise real memory)

Disorders of intelligence

Mental retardation
- Mild mental retardation: IQ 50–70; synonyms include:
  - feeble-minded
  - highgrade defect
  - mild mental subnormality
  - moron
- Moderate mental retardation: IQ 35–49; synonyms include:
  - imbecile
  - moderate mental subnormality
- Severe mental retardation: IQ 20–34; synonyms include:
  - severe mental subnormality
- Profound mental retardation: IQ less than 20; synonyms include:
  - idiocy
  - profound mental subnormality

Dementia
- Global organic impairment of intellectual functioning without impairment of consciousness

Pseudodementia
- Clinically resembles dementia, but not organic in origin
- May be caused by depression

Disorders of body image

Anosognosia
- Lack of awareness of disease

Autotopagnosia
- Inability to name, recognize or point on command to parts of the body

Coenestopathic state
- Localized distortion of body awareness

Distorted awareness of size and shape
- For example, an arm may be felt to be growing larger

Hemisomatognosis
- A limb is felt to be missing
- Also known as hemidepersonalization

Phantom limb
- The continued awareness of a limb or organ that has been removed

Reduplication phenomenon
- Part or all of the body is felt to have been duplicated

Disorders of self-awareness

These are also known as ego disorders, and the following four have been described by Jaspers:

- Disturbance of awareness of self-activity. Types include:
  - depersonalization (the patient feels he or she is altered or not real in some way)
  - derealization (the surroundings do not seem real)
  - loss of emotional resonance
- Disturbance of the immediate awareness of self-unity
- Disturbance of the continuity of self
- Disturbance of the boundaries of the self

Disorders of insight

Insight is not well defined (Lewis) but essentially it refers to the patient's ability to understand the true nature and cause of his or her mental condition.

The questions listed under insight in the previous chapter are a useful way to check the degree of insight present. Note that insight should not simply be said to be present or absent. Rather, the degree of insight should be indicated.

Specimen MCQ

The following may be part of normal experience:

A. Feelings of depersonalization
B. Circumstantiality
C. Audible thoughts
D. Hypnopompic hallucinations
E. Autoscopy

Answers

> A. TRUE Depersonalization sometimes occurs in people who do not have a mental disorder and who are experiencing anxiety, stress, or fatigue

B. TRUE   It can be seen in people without a mental disorder
C. FALSE This is a Schneiderian first rank symptom
D. TRUE
E. TRUE   This phenomenon can occur in normal people who
          are tired and exhausted (Fish)

Bibliography

American Psychiatric Association (1987) *Diagnostic and Statistical Manual of Mental Disorders, Third Edition - Revised (DSM-III-R).* Washington D.C.: American Psychiatric Association.

Berrios, G.E. (1984) Descriptive psychopathology: conceptual and historical aspects. *Psychol. Med.* **14**, 303.

Bleuler, E. (1951) *Dementia Praecox or the Group of Schizophrenias* (trans. J. Zinkin). London: Allen & Unwin.

Cameron, N. (1944) Experimental analysis of schizophrenic thinking. In: Kasanin, J. (editor) *Language and Thought in Schizophrenia.* Berkeley: University of California Press.

Gelder, M., Gath, D. and Mayou, R. (1989) *Oxford Textbook of Psychiatry* 2nd edition. Oxford: Oxford University Press.

Hamilton, M. (editor) (1985) *Fish's Clinical Psychopathology,* 2nd edition. Bristol: Wright.

Jaspers, K. (1962) *General Psychopathology* (trans. M. Hamilton and J. Hoenig). Manchester: Manchester University Press.

Kaplan, H.I. and Sadock, B.J. (editors) (1989) *Comprehensive Textbook of Psychiatry,* 5th edition. Baltimore: Williams and Wilkins.

Kendell, R.E. and Zealley, A.K. (editors) (1988) *Companion to Psychiatric Studies,* 4th edition. Edinburgh: Churchill Livingstone.

Lewis, A. (1934) The psychopathology of insight. *Br. J. Med. Psychol.* **14**, 332.

Schneider, C. (1930) *Psychologie der Schizophrenen* (Psychology of Schizophrenics). Leipzig: Thième.

Schneider, C. (1942) *Die schizophrenen Symptomverbäne* (The Schizophrenic Symptom Groups). Berlin: Springer.

Schneider, K. (1959) *Clinical Psychopathology* (trans. M. Hamilton). New York: Grune & Stratton.

Sims, A.C.P. (1985) *Symptoms in the Mind.* London: Baillière Tindall.

The Royal College of Psychiatrists (1985) *Report to the Court of Electors, The Royal College of Psychiatrists Working Party for Review of the MRCPsych.* London: The Royal College of Psychiatrists.

The Royal College of Psychiatrists (1987) *General Information and Regulations for the MRCPsych Examinations,* 8th revision. London: The Royal College of Psychiatrists.

approximate answers (≠ confabulation)
Ganser ⎰ clouding of consciousness ⎨ concentration↓ attention↓ memory↓
       ⎱ somatic conversion features
       ⎱ pseudohallucinations
? subsequent amnesia.
? dissociative state / malingering

Chapter 8

Dynamic psychopathology

Syllabus requirements

The candidate will be expected to have an awareness of the internal (personality and developmental) and external (environmental) influences which can cause and shape psychopathological phenomena.

This chapter concentrates mainly on giving the reader an introduction to psychotherapeutic concepts.

Introduction

Psychoanalytical theory puts an emphasis on the following:
- Normal mental functioning
- Abnormal mental functioning
- The role of instinctual drives
- Mental conflict
- Mechanisms of defence
- Relationships that one has inside one's mind (internal object relationships)

The mental apparatus is the existence of a stable or relatively stable organization in the individual; in other words, a psychological apparatus involved in both behaviour and subjective experience (dreams and phantasy), and this mental apparatus has a development (oral, anal, genital, Oedipus complex, etc.).

Functions of the mental apparatus

- Control and discharge of excitation
- Defence – the mental apparatus defends against distressing affects and 'incompatible' ideas. The latter are those which were rejected as being unacceptable to the individual's:
  - conscious standards
  - beliefs
  - wishes

- Memory traces – these are laid down by the mental apparatus. Associative links between such traces are created, these links being based on such factors as contemporaneity and similarity of content of events recorded (e.g. birth following a death)
- Attention
- Perception
- Development of the mental apparatus leads to the development of the ego and this is consciousness plus that part of the ego that performs the defence

The unconscious (Freud, 1915)

In the unconscious there is:

- No negation
- Primary process
- Timelessness (reference to time is bound up in unconsciousness)
- Subjection to the pleasure principle
- Censorship (protects consciousness from awareness of instincts which if they were allowed to surface represent a threat; censorship is unconscious)

The severance of unconsciousness and consciousness characterizes a condition of illness. The basic tenet is that behaviour and subjective experience can have unconscious determinants and this applies to normal and abnormal mental functioning. A large part of the mental apparatus functions outside conscious experience. Ideas and feelings can be regarded as existing unconsciously in one form or another.

Censorship

It is appropriate to make use of Sigmund Freud's metaphorical description of the censoring process (1916). 'Let us compare the system of the unconscious to a large entrance hall, in which the mental impulses jostle one another like separate individuals. Adjoining this entrance hall there is a second narrow room, a kind of drawing room, in which consciousness also resides but on the threshold between these two rooms a watchman performs his function; he examines the different mental impulses, acts as a censor, and will not admit them into the drawing room if they displease him. It does not make much difference if the watchman turns away from a particular impulse at the threshold itself or if he pushes it back across the threshold after it has entered the drawing room. If they have already pushed their way forward to the threshold and have been turned back by the watchman then they are inadmissible to the consciousness; we speak of them as *repressed* but even the impulses which the watchman has allowed to cross the threshold are not on that account necessarily conscious as well; they can only become so if they succeed in catching the eye of consciousness. They are therefore justified in calling the second room the system of the *preconscious*.'

Primary process, secondary process

These are two modes of functioning of the mental apparatus. Primary process is characteristic of the unconscious system; secondary process is characteristic of the preconscious and conscious system. The former is about the pleasure principle and the latter about the reality principle.

The study of symptom formation and the analysis of dreams led Freud to recognize a type of mental functioning that was very different from the thought processes which had been the object of traditional psychological observation. Take for example dreaming. Classical psychology has asserted that dreams were characterized by their absence of meaning. Freud maintained they exhibited a constant sliding of meaning, the mechanisms of which are (1) *displacement,* where an apparently insignificant idea comes to be invested with all the psychical depth of meaning and intensity originally attributed to another one, and (2) *condensation,* a process which enables all the meanings and several chains of association to converge on a single idea standing at their point of intersection, e.g. the overdetermination of a symptom. Psychological symptoms have the same structures of condensation and displacement discovered in dreams.

When a primary process is allowed to take its course in connection with elements of preconscious functioning it may appear comic and excite laughter (e.g. a joke).

Characteristics of primary process thinking

- *Timelessness:* concept of time only develops after a period in the mind of a child, in connection to conscious reality, e.g. periodicity or chaos of feeding.
- *Disregard of reality* of the conscious world
- *Psychical reality:* memories of a real event and of imagined experience are not distinguished. Abstract symbols are treated concretely (as in schizophrenia)

- *Absence of contradiction:* opposites have a psychic equivalence. Big and small are the same as far as unconsciousness is concerned
- *Absence of negation:* e.g. 'I remember being beaten by a man who was not like my father', may refer to a repressed memory of being beaten by father

Resistance

This is the name given to everything in words and actions of the analysand that obstructs him or her gaining access to his or her unconscious. By extension, Freud spoke of 'resistance to psychoanalysis' when referring to the hostile attitude towards his discoveries in so far as they exposed unconscious desires and inflicted a 'psychological blow' upon humankind – that we are not so much in charge of ourselves as we imagine.

Resistance was first discovered as an obstacle to the elucidation of symptoms and to the progress of the treatment – it is resistance that seems to bring psychic work to a halt.

At first Freud tried to overcome this obstacle by insistence and persuasion, but then he realized that it was in itself a means of reaching the repressed and uncovering the secrets of neurosis. In fact the forces to be seen at work in resistance and repression are one and the same.

Transference and countertransference

The transference is an unconscious process in which the patient transfers to the therapist feelings, emotions and attitudes that were experienced and/or desired in the patient's childhood, usually in relation to parents and siblings. It can be a passionate demand for love and hate in past relationships between the child and the adult. This is a complex field that includes the unconscious splitting of the therapist into masculine and feminine and locating unconscious affect and thinking of the 'child' part of the patient in relation to the maternal and paternal aspects of the therapist (i.e. oedipal transference). Furthermore, the direction of such a transference can be both positive and negative. Thus, Freud encountered transference in many variations and certainly also in its hidden form, transformed by resistance. The therapist's transference represents on the one hand the most powerful ally but, on the other, in terms of transference's resistance, a therapeutic difficulty.

The countertransference is the therapist's own feelings, emotions and attitudes to his patient. In the treatment mode, the therapist needs to screen out those that are mediated only by the therapist, and take note of those generated in the therapist from emotional contact with the patient. The latter can be an interesting aspect of the patient, e.g. the therapist may have the feelings of the patient as child in relation to the patient enacting the parent. Thus, in the reverse transference, an aspect of the patient is located in the therapist *as a communication*.

The ending of therapy coincides with the breaking of the transference to the therapist, who may be viewed in a more ordinary way without the transference affect from the patient on to the therapist.

Defence mechanisms

These are special mechanisms to protect consciousness by bringing about a form of dissociation of the energy and ideas from consciousness. Defences by their operation may or may not denote pathology. It is normative to have defence mechanisms: the problem can often be conceptualized with the notion that far from having too little in the way of defence mechanisms, the patient can have a defensive structure which is too strong. This may have been necessary for the child to survive physical or psychic attack when small. However, such defensive structure may have created a brick wall around that person's relationships and affects such that it is inappropriate in the adult and for the adult's relationships.

Repression

Repression is the basic defence. It is pushing away (*verdrangung*) of unacceptable ideas and emotions, relegating them to the unconscious. If it is successful no trace of the distressing idea or feeling remains in consciousness but a quantity of affective excitation remains, e.g. a person having forgotten and being unable to recall something which he or she had read (and normally expected to remember) because the content of a particular passage aroused unpalatable memories of past sexual events. These memories and emotions give rise to the affective reaction of repugnance and the memories, affects and associated contents of what was recently read were 'pushed away' from consciousness, i.e. repressed.

Reaction formation

Psychological attitude diametrically opposed to an oppressed wish and constituted as a reaction against it, e.g. bashfulness, countering exhibitionist tendencies. It is often seen in obsessional character traits.

Isolation

Characteristic of obsessional neurosis, isolating thoughts and behaviour so that links with other thoughts or the rest of life is broken, e.g. pauses in train of thought, formulae, rituals, etc.

Undoing (what has been done)

The subject makes an attempt to cause past thoughts, words, gestures, or actions not to have occurred, i.e. the compulsion of magic especially in obsessional neurotics.

Projection

Qualities, feelings, wishes (or even objects) which the subject refuses to recognize or rejects in himself or herself and which are located in another person or thing.

Projective identification (Klein)

A mode of defence in which the subject not only sees the other person as possessing aspects of the self which the subject has repressed, but actually constrains the other person to 'take on' those aspects. It is therefore a truly 'interperson' defence and can often be detected by the therapist through his or her countertransference.

Introjection (Ferenzci)

In phantasy the subject transposes objects and their qualities from their 'outside' to the 'inside' of himself or herself. This is close to incorporation and identification e.g. 'good enough to eat'.

Turning against the self

Process whereby the instinct replaces an independent object by the subject's own self (i.e. it concerns the object).

Reversal into the opposite

Aim of the instinct is transferred into its opposite in the transition from activity to passivity, i.e. it concerns the aim, e.g. sadism/masochism, voyeurism/exhibitionism.

Rationalization (Jones)

An attempt to explain in a logically consistent or ethically acceptable way, ideas, thoughts and feelings whose true motive is not perceived. This is very common in everyday life and is a secondary defence, camouflaging the various factors in defensive conflict. It can be seen operating in delusional symptoms to account 'as if' rationally, for bizarre ideas.

Sublimation

Process to account for human activities which have no apparent connection with sexuality but which are assumed to be motivated with the force of a sexual instinct, e.g. artistic creation and intellectual enquiry (the quest of a child for knowledge, to know, to ascertain how a baby is made).

Idealization

The object's qualities are elevated to the point of perfection.

Dreams, daydreams, symptoms, character traits, works of art and other forms of behaviour and experience are regarded as compromise formations between the instinctual wish and all the forces which oppose instinctual gratification.

Regression

Transition, under times of stress and threat, to moods of expression and functioning that are on a lower level of complexity. Moving from an adult to a childlike functioning.

There is regression from adult forms of sexuality to infantile ones and this is not necessarily associated with illness, as everyone has such capacities. Malignant regression is seen when a patient collapses from a general capacity to function as an adult into someone that has to be fed, bathed, soothed and cared for, with little inclination to do that for themselves.

Examination of the clinical relationship

Examination of the clinical relationship between the doctor and his (or her) patient provides valuable clues in understanding the psychodynamic psychopathology. A patient can only relate to another in the manner he (or she) undertakes any of his relationships, in his own idiosyncratic ways. This is developed from the way each of us has imbibed our loves and hates, likes and dislikes, as we have grown up in relation to our parents, siblings and teachers, etc. The initial way the patient relates to the other is the terrain the doctor can explore in the clinical interview.

The handling of the opening of the clinical interview and its initial resistances can set the tone for the whole of what follows. Prior to entering the clinic, the patient usually has had contact by way of a letter and an appointment time. Of course the general practitioner may also have directed the patient's thoughts and feelings towards what may happen. These will inevitably stimulate fantasies of what may happen in the psychiatric interview, as well as expectation and hope.

The patient enters the consulting room and is invited to sit in a chair. At once the doctor has begun observing. It is important to notice how the patient is dressed, his expression and whether a handshake is proffered. The initial effect that the person has on us has already made an impression in the mind of the interviewer, which can then be begun to be matched with the content of the interview. The patient may step into the room with a smiling bonhomie as if meeting a friend for a drink. Or the patient may shrink as far away as possible from the start of the interview.

It should be noticed how the patient sits and the general ambience of the patient in the setting of the room. It would be normal for anyone to have some level of anxiety about seeing a new doctor for an appointment which may well be a significant event in that person's life. If the patient is devoid of anxiety then it is important that this is recognized and an internal question asked.

Often the patient arrives with expectations of what will happen and may work very hard to realize such fantasies. For instance, it is very common to expect to be asked many questions by the doctor. This, after all, is often how general practitioners work, and how the patient has usually been treated by doctors in the past. At this point, Michael Balint's dictum, 'if you ask a question you get an answer and nothing else', is very apposite. It is usually true that the patient has standard replies already in his mind, often, but not always, consciously, to the questions he is expecting to be asked. The idea that he, the patient, should begin to reveal himself, to talk about himself and what is on his mind, may well be a unique experience. Although people ask for consultations with psychiatrists in order to begin to try and make sense of their thoughts and feelings, it also of course arouses anxiety, and often intense resistance.

The patient is confronted with a quiet setting which is the room, two chairs where he and the psychiatrist sit, and time to begin to try and look at that person's world and their interpersonal difficulties. It would seem that some sort of special conditions have been established to allow the patient to give expression to himself. However, it is this very space that often arouses resistance, anger and hostility.

Having looked, the psychiatrist must also listen very intently. It is important not just to listen to the content, but also to be aware of the affect of the patient that embellishes the content, and the context that the patient weaves in the telling of the story. To further complicate matters, whatever affect the patient seems to be investing in his story, the doctor also has feelings, which may or may not be stirred. It is an interesting clinical phenomenon when a receptive psychiatrist is in the presence of a patient who seems to be telling a very harrowing story and is in tears and despair, which, however, leaves the psychiatrist untouched and unmoved. It could well behove the psychiatrist to take account of such phenomena in order to differentiate between real sadness and real psychic pain from the camouflage of crocodile tears. To enable the psychiatrist to manage such careful balancing, he must be in a neutral state of mind. By this is meant that he should neither be for nor against his patient, but in a state of suspension, waiting to see the impact of the patient's thoughts and feelings on the psychiatrist. With experience the psychiatrist will begin to gauge and have a knowledge of how the patient is making use of him.

There is no reason at all to think that every patient in every clinical examination with a psychiatrist is only going to tell the truth. It is quite common for some people to blame others for their own difficulties and inadequacies in life. Such people may derive much benefit in attempting to gain a psychiatrist to be on their side against, for instance, a spouse or another member of the family. This may well appease in the heat of the moment, but in the long-term management it may really be just an avoidance of underlying traits.

Another way in which the doctor's own feelings of the clinical interview are often of great importance is in the presence of manic patients. Here the phenomenon of the patient being extremely hilarious is often seen and, notwithstanding the severity of the psychopathology, a doctor finds himself laughing uproarously at yet another enormously funny story. This is another interesting psychodynamic paradox in which a tragedy of the other side of the patient's mania, his depressive state, is split off from the clinical interview and instead the patient unconsciously gets a psychiatrist to collude in the hilarity, as opposed to the sadness. As in the earlier examples, the psychiatrist can keep an observing ego inside himself, seeing what is going on in the clinical relationship. He may be left with enough presence of mind to make sense of the phenomenon that is engaging him.

To return to the balance between content and context: this is a crucial parameter. You may well be in the presence of a patient who is telling the contents of a story very fully and intellectually, and yet if you look at the context of the telling you are left wondering where the emotions of the patient are. The psychiatrist can then begin to perceive in such an imbalance that the affect is missing and can then ask the internal question why and where has it gone and what is it? If on listening to the story you have a sense that any ordinary person might have a particular feeling such as anger about the circumstances that have occurred to the patient, it may well be worth-while asking the patient why they are not making any mention of a particular affect such as anger or sadness, for instance. The value of this for the patient is that the emotional side of the patient, which may be in the grip of an intellectual understanding only, will sense that the psychiatrist is able to listen to the totality of the experience trying to be conveyed including what is being left out.

The ending of the clinical interview

Care needs to be given to how the ending of the clinical interview is achieved. The psychiatrist may have gathered enough information to be at a point of ending the clinical interview when the patient is not as ready as the doctor. Having opened up the patient's private world and emotional state it can be quite cruel to not attend to the 'putting back together again' of the patient prior to his leaving the interview. In this area tact is needed. For instance, intention to finish the interview in a few minutes can be signalled; this will give the patient warning, rather than to abruptly curtail something which the patient may well find of great intimacy. It is often useful to inquire what the patient has made of the interview.

At this point in the clinical interview the ego strength of the patient can also be examined; whether they can bear to separate and continue managing for themselves, or whether there ensues a more primitive state of mind in which there is much importuning of the doctor or adhesiveness such that it may be unbearable for the patient to stop even taking their eyes off the doctor. Again, the psychiatrist is able to make use of this part of the clinical interview in a valuable way to glean fragments of understanding about the patient's capacities for ending, which may be of great use, in time, in planning the patient's ending in treatment, either as an outpatient or inpatient.

It is also a vital part of the interview that the anxiety that the psychiatrist feels within himself about the dangerousness of leaving the patient alone can often be most marked if it has not appeared before in the interview. This may be the point where the psychiatrist can really obtain a feel of the anxiety of suicidalness or murderousness imparted by the patient to his doctor.

The patient in the setting of the ward

By observing the relationships that the patient encloses himself within the ward the expression of his internal relationships can be gauged. Thus some patients will attempt to lead others whilst others expect to be lead. Some will embellish their histories to others whilst some will be totally silent and alone. It is common for certain types of patients to engage in splitting the staff up into good and bad, with a transference into staff members of the patient's view of their own family atmosphere. Some staff are taken in by the direction of the patient's positiveness towards them, as if they really were 'the only person I could talk to'. This splitting of the field then leaves other staff members to be perceived as the awful bad mendacious characters in the play that the patient is directing on the ward. Again, with the observing ego, taking in the whole field, the psychiatrist can view the range of emotional ties in the staff, both positive and negative, as being a product of all aspects of the patient. This is clinically more sound than taking cognizance of only a 'good' aspect of the personality. The totality of the patient needs to be seen and made sense of by the psychiatrist.

Very often the splits in the ward can be seen to be made by the patient as if they are between the nurses versus the doctors or senior staff versus junior staff. It is important for the psychiatrist to recognize such divisive atmospheres surrounding a particular patient as being the internal struggles inside that patient's unconscious self, which is then projected into various characters called the ward staff. What follows from this perception by the psychiatrist will in due course be a capacity to assimilate thoughts about the atmosphere and intensity of the patient's internal object relationships, and be able to make a comment that makes sense to the patient about a totality of the aspects of their struggles in relation to themselves and other people. (This is not being dealt with in this book as it goes beyond its brief.)

In summary:

- The psychiatrist needs to note his own emotional reaction towards his patient
- The psychiatrist's affect is a clue to the emotional life of his patient

- This may be congruent with the affect the patient expresses or separate
- If the latter it may mean a more complex emotional state in the patient who is in touch with some of his own emotions and yet projecting other affect into the doctor
- It is helpful if the psychiatrist takes a neutral amoralistic stance towards his patient
- The psychiatrist needs to be curious. The psychiatrist can often evaluate other aspects of the totality of the patient's system of relationships by interviewing others in the family and/or seeing the patient in a ward setting

The sexual life of the patient

Patients when having an interview with the psychiatrist invariably expect their sexual life to be evaluated. If the psychiatrist does not ask about this part of his patient's life in an ordinary way, similar to how a general practitioner may examine the whole of his patient's body, the patient might well feel that the psychiatrist is too shy and embarrassed, which inevitably has clinical consequences of lack of confidence in the doctor. This area of the mental health and illness of the patient should be approached in an ordinary matter-of-fact way that one would use to examine any other part of the patient's psyche-soma. (This of course may require considerable personal work by the psychiatrist in evaluating his own sexual state of mind.)

The way in which a person values and utilizes their sexual life in all its various meanings gives the psychiatrist useful data to understand the quality of relationships and in particular its affective qualities. In the interview such data can be compared with the developmental history of how the child perceived himself to have been brought up, as well as his connections to the present symptomatology in particular difficulties of relationships that exist beneath the broad symptoms.

If you ask yourself the question 'What is sexual?', a whole range of ideas can spring to mind, viz.:

- Intercourse between male and female
- Reproduction
- Childbirth
- Pleasure in one's own body
- Kissing
- Masturbation
- Perversion

Kissing may not be seen to be perverse, but many couples are disgusted at the notion of sharing a toothbrush!

Freud postulated the innate bisexuality of men and women. Thus hysterical symptoms are an expression on the one hand of a masculine unconscious phantasy, and on the other hand of a feminine one. The idea of masculinity and femininity being part of men and women leads to a rich tapestry of the various metaphors and meanings construed in a relationship.

A *perversion* is defined (in the *Shorter Oxford English Dictionary*) as a turning aside from the truth – it is this aspect of sexuality that it is useful to explore clinically, as a turning aside from a truth about oneself can be enmeshed in the details of sexual lives.

Freud (in *Three Essays on Sexuality,* 1905) divided perversion into:

1. Those in which a sexual object has been altered
2. Those in which the sexual aim has been altered

In the first category the vagina is exchanged, by the man, for the mouth, anus, etc. so that sexuality can be linked to the gastrointestinal tract, or exchanged for a foot, hair or piece of clothing (the fetish object); an extreme variety being the necrophiliac who exchanges a live sexual object for a corpse.

In the second category the aim is not intercourse per se, but voyeurism/exhibitionism or sadism/masochism.

The systematic study of the perversions was topical when Freud was beginning to work out his theory of sexuality (Krafft-Ebing's *Psychopathia Sexualis* dating from 1893 and Havelock Ellis' *Studies in the Psychology of Sex* 1897). The 'normal' sexual act can be defined as coitus with a person of the opposite sex, and is directed towards the achievement of orgasm by means of genital penetration. Perversion can be defined as existing where the orgasm is reached with other sexual objects (homosexuality, paedophilia, bestiality, etc.), or through other regions of the body (anal coitus, etc.). Where the orgasm is subordinated absolutely to certain extrinsic conditions, these may even be sufficient in themselves to bring about sexual pleasure (fetishism, transvestism, voyeurism, exhibitionism and sadomasochism). In psychoanalysis 'perversion' has a meaning in terms of the whole psychosexual behaviour that accompanies such atypical means of obtaining sexual pleasure, and investigating it with a patient will provide information on the atmosphere of the relationships in that person's life (past as well as present).

By clinically examining the sexual life of the patient, both in reality and in their imaginative ideas, the psychiatrist is able to palpate more of the details and directions of the emotional structure of mental life. If the psychiatrist is keen, with a patient who is interested, the developmental line can be examined, viz.:

Dynamic life stages	Possible psychopathological positions
Mother's feeding relationship with the infant	The development of a sense of trust A child feeling it was or was not loved The first love object is the breast – this acts as a template for future relationships To quote Freud 'the finding of an object is the refinding of the first object' (1905)
How weaning was achieved	With mutuality between mother and child or in mother's interest alone This may leave the child with a template for emotional instability and depression
The child's perception of the parental relationship	Oedipal relationships – the child has a notion of whether his parents are a psychosexual couple or whether there is distance and separation psychically
Childhood sexual play – autoerotic	Narcissistic in character structure Excitation without discharge (i.e. no orgasm)
In relationship to other children	Ability to relate to friends of both sexes Movement towards heterosexuality Incest Bedwetting School refusal

Adolescence	Capacity for orgasm
Coming to terms with a genital body	Incest
How this is viewed by parents who can have pleasure or negativity about such transitions	Compulsive masturbation that replaces thinking and learning
Adult sexuality	Capacity for concern with the other
	Adult genitality
	Perversion
Marriage	The atmosphere of marital life
	The use and/or abuse of the partner
	Loving and hating
Parenthood	How the patient is the same as or different from how they perceive their own parents to be towards themselves as they were growing up
	The possibility of transgenerational pathology by doing to one's own children what was inflicted on oneself when young, e.g. identification with the aggressor (A. Freud)
	Stillbirths and terminations of pregnancy, mourning
Middle age	Mid-life crisis
Retirement	Problems of children reaching adulthood and leaving home
Loss of job	
Problems of ageing	
Loss of self-esteem	Capacity to mourn for others and in anticipation of self
Death	Capacity to mourn may now be seen to link with the handling of the mourning in the early relationship with the mother and the loss of the first object, the breast

Specimen MCQ

The unconscious:

A. Contains internal objects
B. Is timeless
C. Is full of resistance
D. Contains childhood wishes that have become fixated
E. Tests reality

Answers

A. TRUE
B. TRUE
C. FALSE Resistance is the name given to everything in words and actions of the analysand that obstructs his gaining access to his unconscious
D. TRUE
E. FALSE Reality testing is a process postulated by Sigmund Freud to distinguish stimuli originating in the outside world from the internal world, and to forestall possible confusion between what one perceives and what is only imagined

Bibliography

Ellis, H. (1901) *Studies in the Psychology of Sex,* Vol. 2. *Sexual inversion.* Philadelphia: Davis.
Ellis, H. (1928) *Studies in the Psychology of Sex,* Vol. 7. *Eonism and other supplementary Studies.* Philadelphia: Davis.
Freeman, T. (1988) *The Psychoanalyst and Psychiatry.* London: Karnac.
Freud, A. (1936) *The Ego and the Mechanisms of Defence.* London: Hogarth Press.
Freud, S. (1986) *The Essentials of Psychoanalysis.* Harmondsworth: Pelican Books.
Kaplan, H.I. and Sadock, B.J. (editors) (1989) *Comprehensive Textbook of Psychiatry,* 5th edition. Baltimore: Williams and Wilkins.
Krafft-Ebing, R. (1924) *Psychopathic Sexuality with Special Reference to Contrary Sexual Instinct.* Authorized translation of the 7th German edition. Philadelphia: C.G. Chaddock.
Laplanche J. and Pontalis J. B. (1973) *The Language of Psychoanalysis.* London: Hogarth Press.
Sandler, J., Dare, C. and Holder, A. (1988) *The Patient and the Analyst.* London: Hogarth Press.
The Royal College of Psychiatrists (1985) *Report to the Court of Electors, The Royal College of Psychiatrists Working Party for Review of the MRCPsych.* London: The Royal College of Psychiatrists.
The Royal College of Psychiatrists (1987) *General Information and Regulations for the MRCPsych Examinations,* 8th revision. London: The Royal College of Psychiatrists.

Chapter 9
Classification

Syllabus requirements

The candidate will be expected to have an understanding of the principles underlying the classification of psychiatric phenomena into syndromes.

The concept of mental illness

Illnesses in general medicine may be classified on the basis of:

- Aetiology
- Structural pathology
- Symptoms (for example migraine)

Most general medical conditions can be classified under the first two systems. However, in psychiatry, only a few conditions can be classified on the basis of aetiology or pathology, for example, general paralysis of the insane. The majority have to be classified by the third system shown above. This is likely to change in the future with the increasing understanding of aetiology and pathology afforded by molecular neurobiological techniques.

Defining mental illness has proved to be difficult. By analogy with general medicine, one could define it as:

- The absence of health
- The presence of suffering
- A pathological process

Absence of health

The question then arises as to the definition of the term health. The World Health Organisation defined health as 'a state of complete physical, mental and social well-being, and not merely the absence of disease or infirmity'.

This definition of health has been criticized as being overinclusive and meaningless (Lewis).

The presence of suffering

This definition might not apply, for example, to a manic patient who has an intense feeling of well-being.

Pathological process

Szasz has argued that illness can only be defined in terms of pathology which can be physically demonstrated. He has argued that mental illness is a myth used by society.

A widening of the concept of pathology to include, for example, genetics, would tend to negate the arguments of Szasz and others, by recognizing pathological processes at work in many mental illnesses.

With the advent of the application of molecular genetic and molecular biological techniques to mental illnesses, it may be possible in the future to classify many more mental illnesses by 'pathology'.

Socially deviant behaviour

Lewis and Wooton have argued against using this criterion to define mental illnesses. Such a definition is clearly open to political abuse in certain countries.

Psychopathology

Lewis argued in favour of defining mental illness in terms of psychopathology.

Principles of psychiatric classification

Mental illnesses are usually considered to:

- Occur following a period of normal adult functioning
- Have a recognizable onset

Therefore, the following disorders are usually separated from mental illness:

- Mental retardation (on the grounds that this is present continuously from birth or childhood)
- Personality disorder (on the grounds that this is present continuously from adolescence)

Mental illnesses are usually then divided into psychoses and neuroses:

- Psychoses can be organic or functional
- They are difficult to define but are usually said to be characterized by symptoms such as delusions, hallucinations and lack of insight
- The neuroses include obsessive compulsive disorders, anxiety disorders, hysterical disorders and hypochondriasis
- Other disorders not included above may be classified separately, e.g. sexual disorders (see below)

Objections have been raised to the use of diagnoses and classification systems in psychiatry. This is a large area which is unlikely to be examined in detail in the MRCPsych Part I Examination. Therefore, further details are not given here, but the interested reader is referred to the bibliography at the end of the chapter.

Symptoms and diagnoses
Only a minority of mental illnesses have pathognomonic symptoms. However, each illness can be seen as a group of symptoms or a syndrome. 'Phenomenological symptoms' in a given patient are then classified as being part of a given psychiatric classification by having the latter defined in terms of the presence of some or most of a group of symptoms (rather than by the presence of one pathognomonic symptom). According to Kendell: 'In the jargon of nosology the psychiatric illnesses are polythetic rather than monothetic.'

Categorical classification

This is the traditional way in which psychiatric disorders have been classified.

Advantages
Kendell has summarized the advantages of categories over dimensions:

- Greater familiarity
- Easier to understand, remember and use
- Provide a prelude to action (e.g. treatment)
- They do not strain the resources of a largely innumerate profession

Hierarchy
A hierarchy is often used when more than one diagnosis is made for a patient at a given time. For example, conventionally, in the following list a diagnosis takes precedence over those below it:

- Organic psychosis
- Functional psychosis
- Neurosis

Foulds' hierarchical classification system has 4 classes and 12 categories. In order of increasing priority, the classes are:

Class 1: dysthymic states
Class 2: neurotic symptoms
Class 3: 'integrated delusions'
Class 4: 'delusions of disintegration'

A high priority class can be accompanied by symptoms of a lower class priority, but only the former is diagnosed.

ICD-9
The World Health Organization's 1978 *Ninth Revision of the International Classification of Diseases* (Glossary of Mental Disorders and Guide to their Classification) is a categorical classification which contains the following main diagnostic groups:

	ICD-9 code
Organic psychotic conditions	
Senile and presenile organic psychotic conditions	290
Alcoholic psychoses	291
Drug psychoses	292
Transient organic psychotic conditions	293
Other organic psychotic conditions (chronic)	294
Other psychoses	
Schizophrenic psychoses	295
Affective psychoses	296
Paranoid states	297
Other non-organic psychoses	298
Psychoses with origin specific to childhood	299
Neurotic disorders, personality disorders and other non-psychotic mental disorders	
Neurotic disorders	300
Personality disorders	301
Sexual deviations and disorders	302
Alcohol dependence syndrome	303
Drug dependence	304

Non-categorical classification

Dimensional approach
Patients are assigned to a position on at least one axis or
dimension. It has been strongly supported by Eysenck (see
below).

Advantages   Kendell has summarized the advantages of dimensions over categories:

- More information is conveyed
- There is greater flexibility
- The presence of unproven qualitative differences between
  different subpopulation members is not implied
- Artificial boundaries are not imposed and the observer's
  perception of individuals lying near boundaries between
  adjacent categories is not distorted

Eysenck's dimensional approach   Arguing strongly against categorical classification, Eysenck has proposed a three-dimensional
system:

- Neuroticism
- Psychoticism
- Introversion/extraversion

Multiaxial approach
In this approach at least two sets of information are coded separately (see below). One of the most widely used multiaxial classification systems is the American Psychiatric Association's *Diagnostic and Statistical Manual of Mental Disorders,* third edition – revised (DSM-III-R). This was published in 1987, replacing the 1980 DSM-III, which was also a multiaxial classification system.

DSM-III-R   There are five axes:

Axis I – Clinical syndromes
        – V codes (for conditions not attributable to a mental disorder that are a focus of attention or treatment)
Axis II – Developmental disorders
        – Personality disorders
Axis III – Physical disorders and conditions
Axis IV – Severity of psychosocial stressors
Axis V – Global assessment of functioning

The main Axis I categories and codes are:

Disorders usually first evident in infancy, childhood, or adolescence

Disruptive behaviour disorders	312, 313, 314
Anxiety disorders of childhood or adolescence	309, 313
Eating disorders	307
Gender identity disorders	302
Tic disorders	307
Elimination disorders	307
Speech disorders not elsewhere classified	307
Other disorders of infancy, childhood, or adolescence	307, 313, 314

Organic mental disorders

Dementias arising in the senium and presenium	290
Psychoactive substance-induced organic mental disorders	291, 292, 303, 305
Organic mental disorders associated with Axis III physical disorders or conditions, or whose aetiology is unknown	293, 294, 310

Psychoactive substance use disorders	304, 305
Schizophrenia	295
Delusional (paranoid) disorder	297
Psychotic disorders not elsewhere classified	295, 297, 298

Mood disorders
    Bipolar disorders   296, 301
    Depressive disorders   296, 300, 311
Anxiety disorders (or anxiety and phobic neurosis)   300, 309
Somatoform disorders   300, 307
Dissociative disorders (or hysterical neuroses,
dissociative type)   300
Sexual disorders
    Paraphilias   302
    Sexual dysfunctions   302, 306
    Other sexual disorders   302

Sleep disorders
    Dyssomnias   307, 780
    Parasomnias   307

Factitious disorders   300, 301
Impulse control disorders not elsewhere classified   312
Adjustment disorder   309
Psychological factors affecting physical condition   316
V codes for conditions not attributable to a mental
disorder that are a focus of attention or treatment
                                        V15, V61, V62, V65, V71

The main Axis II categories and codes are:

Disorders usually first evident in infancy, childhood,
or adolescence
    Mental retardation   317–319
    Pervasive developmental disorders   299
    Specific developmental disorders   315
    Other developmental disorders   315
Personality disorders

    Cluster A   301
    Cluster B   301
    Cluster C   301

V40.00 (Borderline intellectual functioning) is also coded on axis
II

Psychodynamic nosology

Neurosis

A neurosis is a psychogenic manifestation in which symptoms are
symbolic expressions of psychic conflict whose origin lies in the

childhood history. Such symptoms constitute a compromise between wishes and defence.

Anxiety neurosis
Predominance of anxiety with the chronic expectation of it happening again. Anxiety attacks may be psychological or somatic (as in hyperventilation). The point of the expectation of it happening again is indicative that it may already have happened in the past and in particular in the early developmental history of the patient. Somatic equivalents of anxiety include features of autonomic hyperactivity (e.g. diarrhoea), features caused by hyperventilation (e.g. paraesthesiae) and features caused by increased muscle tension (e.g. chest pain). Phobic symptoms are where the affect of anxiousness is bound to a particular idea. Dynamically the same way of understanding the components of a dream via condensation and displacement allow the elucidation of such symptomatology in the psyche-soma.

Conversion hysteria
Conversion of symptoms is the mechanism which operates in hysteria where there is a deflection of psychical conflict through somatic symptoms which may be either of a motor nature, e.g. paralysis, or a sensory one, e.g. anaesthesia and pain. The conversion symptoms are typically symbolic of repressed ideas expressed through the medium of the body. Hence the field of psychosomatics.

Obsessional neurosis
The psychic conflict is expressed through symptoms described as obsessive–compulsive ideas, compulsions towards undesirable acts, and struggles against these thoughts. These include rituals. Also, there is an attack on thinking which is seen with ruminations and doubts which prevent action. Dynamically there is a displacement of affect on to ideas that are struggled with away from the original conflict. Thus obsessions and rituals and circular ruminative thoughts defend against particular thoughts and feelings that are too painful to be known, usually in the area of hate.

The character neurosis
This is a particular sort of neurosis in which the conflict, instead of having identifiable symptoms, is seen as character traits, modes of behaviour or the totality of a particular personality. This is most clearly seen with the presentation of patients with problems in

their relationships and questioning their identity. Much psychoanalysis these days is in the area of character analysis (after Reich, 1933) in which the defensive structure surrounding the particular object relationships of the individual are examined in terms of developmental history and present difficulties of living in the world with the vicissitudes of relationships.

Psychosis

Psychosis is a disturbance in the relationship between the ego and the external world. As well as delusions of persecution, Freud placed erotomania, delusional jealousy and delusions of grandeur under the heading of paranoia. Objects may be split into good idealized objects which provide unlimited immediate and everlasting gratification, and these defend against persecutory anxiety. The other half of the picture is that the bad object is a terrifying persecutor that exposes its owner to threats of destruction. As a means of defence the ego splits itself and uses the mental mechanisms of denial as well as omnipotent control.

Depression and mania

Experiences which precipitate depression represent either a loss of self-esteem or loss of supplies which one had hoped would be available. In ordinary life these would be various failures, loss of money, disappointment in love, the death of a loved person or tasks which make somebody feel objectively or subjectively aware of their inferiority. The model for how one deals with loss later in life can be found in how it was dealt with early on. The earliest template is the loss of the breast. Ordinary grief involves looking at a vast number of memories that link a person to the lost object, and each of these memories contains affect. The time this takes is the work of mourning and must last at least until the first anniversary, and usually beyond.

In depressive psychopathology the self-reproaches can be of a delusional nature. Now the depressed patient is concerned that he is worthless and instead of having lost an object he becomes as worthless as what has been lost itself (as Freud puts it, 'The shadow of the object has fallen on the ego'). Dynamically, the suicidal attempt always contains a murderous attack that then is contained by directing it against the self rather than the other.

In mania the other side of the ambivalence is shown with a marked increase in self-esteem. In depression the ego can be perceived as entirely powerless and the superego omnipotent, whereas in mania the ego has regained omnipotence and triumphs.

In mania the ego has managed to free itself from the pressure of the superego and terminated its conflict with the shadow of the lost object and then seems to 'celebrate' such a happening.

Specimen MCQ

The presence of the following in a patient would strongly suggest that he or she is suffering from a psychotic illness:

A. Thought broadcasting
B. Transvestism
C. Audible thoughts
D. Hypnagogic hallucinations
E. Obsessional thoughts

Answers

A. TRUE This is a Schneiderian first rank symptom
B. FALSE Transvestism is a form of sexual deviation in which sexual pleasure is derived from dressing in the clothes of the opposite gender
C. TRUE This is a Schneiderian first rank symptom
D. FALSE Although these are hallucinations, and the latter are said to be a characteristic feature of psychoses, hypnagogic hallucinations often occur as part of normal experience, and are therefore not strongly suggestive of psychosis
E. FALSE These are classed as neuroses

Bibliography

American Psychiatric Association (1980) *Diagnostic and Statistical Manual of Mental Disorders, Third Edition (DSM-III).* Washington D.C.: American Psychiatric Association.

American Psychiatric Association (1987) *Diagnostic and Statistical Manual of Mental Disorders, Third Edition–Revised (DSM-III-R).* Washington D.C.: American Psychiatric Association.

Eysenck H.J. (editor) (1960) *Handbook of Abnormal Psychology: An Experimental Approach.* London: Pitman.

Eysenck H.J. (1976) *The Learning Theory Model of Neurosis: A New Approach.* Behaviour Research and Therapy 14, 251-267.

Freeman, T. (1988) *The Psychoanalyst and Psychiatry.* London: Karnac.

Freud, S. (1986) *The Essentials of Psychoanalysis.* Harmondsworth: Pelican Books.

Gelder, M., Gath, D. and Mayou, R. (1989) *Oxford Textbook of Psychiatry.* 2nd edition. Oxford: Oxford University Press.

Kaplan, H.I. and Sadock, B.J. (editors) (1989) *Comprehensive Textbook of Psychiatry,* 5th edition. Baltimore: Williams and Wilkins.

158   Classification

Kendell, R.E. (1975) *The Role of Diagnosis in Psychiatry*. Oxford: Blackwell Scientific.

Kendell, R.E. and Zealley, A.K. (editors) (1988) *Companion to Psychiatric Studies*, 4th edition. Edinburgh: Churchill Livingstone.

Laplanche J. and Pontalis J. B. (1973) *The Language of Psychoanalysis*. London: Hogarth Press.

Lewis, A.J. (1953) Health as a social concept. *British Journal of Sociology* **4**, 109–124.

Roth, M. (1976) Schizophrenia and the theories of Thomas Szasz. *British Journal of Psychiatry* **129**, 317–326.

Roth, M. and Kroll, J. (1986) *The Reality of Mental Illness*. Cambridge: Cambridge University Press.

Sandler, J., Dare, C. and Holder, A. (1988) *The Patient and the Analyst*. London: Hogarth Press

Szasz, T. (1976) Schizophrenia: the sacred symbol of psychiatry. *British Journal of Psychiatry* **129**, 308–316.

The Royal College of Psychiatrists (1985) *Report to the Court of Electors, The Royal College of Psychiatrists Working Party for Review of the MRCPsych*. London: The Royal College of Psychiatrists.

The Royal College of Psychiatrists (1987) *General Information and Regulations for the MRCPsych examinations*, 8th revision. London: The Royal College of Psychiatrists.

World Health Organisation (1978) *Mental Disorders: Glossary and Guide to their Classification in Accordance with the Ninth Revision of the International Classification of Diseases (ICD-9)*. World Health Organisation, Geneva.

Index